Healthy & Free

Study Guide

DESTINY IMAGE BOOKS BY BENI JOHNSON

The Happy Intercessor

The Joy of Intercession

Beautiful One (with Heidi Baker et al)

Experiencing the Heavenly Realm (with Judy Franklin)

Walking in the Supernatural (with Bill Johnson et al)

Healthy & Free

Study Guide

A JOURNEY TO WELLNESS FOR YOUR BODY, SOUL, AND SPIRIT

Beni Johnson

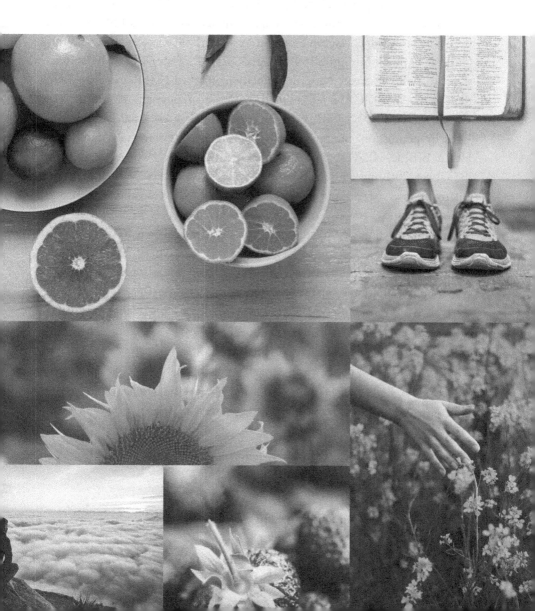

DESTINY IMAGE® PUBLISHERS, INC.

P.O. Box 310, Shippensburg, PA 17257-0310

"Promoting Inspired Lives."

This book and all other Destiny Image and Destiny Image Fiction books are available at Christian bookstores and distributors worldwide.

Cover design by Bethel Media

For more information on foreign distributors, call 717-532-3040.

Reach us on the Internet: www.destinyimage.com.

ISBN 13 TP: 978-0-7684-0796-9

For Worldwide Distribution, Printed in the U.S.A.

3 4 5 6 7 8 / 20 19 18 17

Contents

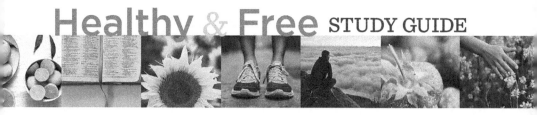

Introduction

I firmly believe that the body of Christ—the Church—should be the healthiest community of people on the planet. Unfortunately, this has often been the opposite. We have done well to invest in our spiritual lives, only to neglect the physical temple that God has arranged for His Spirit to dwell in on earth—our human bodies! The apostle Paul really meant it when he wrote that our "bodies are temples of the Holy Spirit" (1 Cor. 6:19 NIV).

Healthy and Free is designed to take you on a journey to wholeness—body, soul, and spirit. This is *not* intended to be the final word on exercise, nutrition, or any other health-related topic. Instead, the book and curriculum are being presented to you with *one very clear* purpose: To help get you started on your personal journey!

Once you get started on *your journey*, we have listed many different resources that will help you along the way (these are presented in the *Healthy and Free* book). The problem for so many of us is that we don't know where to *start*. It can feel daunting, especially if you feel like you have a long way to go toward reaching your desired health goals.

Right now, don't focus so much on how long you think it will take to get where you need to be. The most important things you can do by going on the *Healthy and Free* journey are as follows:

- Find your why and get a vision for why it's important for you to begin a journey toward health and wholeness.

- Get started and begin to take daily baby steps toward your goal. Don't overwhelm yourself—the key is starting wherever you are right now!

- See beyond a diet…and recognize that *Healthy and Free* is not about a fad or even a season where you eat a certain way (only to go back to "normal"); this journey is about beginning some new normals in your life.

And remember, the journey to becoming *Healthy and Free* is uniquely yours! I am here to come alongside you to help jumpstart this great adventure into wholeness. Take it day by day, one step at a time.

To your health!

Beni Johnson

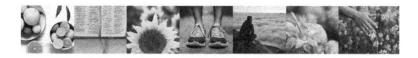

How to Use This Curriculum

Here are a few ways that you can go through the *Healthy and Free* sessions:

As a Small Group

You can join together with a few friends, or officially join/start a small group out of your church. This would require a group leader/host and a host venue.

As a Discipleship Class

You could go through these sessions as a discipleship class at your church. This would require a class leader/instruction and a venue—most likely, a church.

As an Individual Journey

You could also go through these eight sessions as an individual journey, engaging the study guide exercises yourself and watching the video sessions as you make your way through the curriculum.

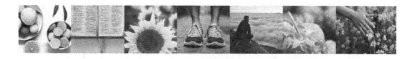

Format of Curriculum

You will go through one video session each week.

During your class/group meeting, you will watch the designated video session, dialogue about what you learned, and then participate in an activation exercise.

The goal for each session is to give you tools that will help you start making new health choices—in a way that is conducive to your lifestyle. Many who go through these sessions will be confronted with the need for significant lifestyle changes. While the wake-up call is always necessary, too many of us engage it incorrectly. A wake-up call is not cause to immediately rush out and try to make (in your own strength) a dramatic health overhaul. If you try this, you will be disappointed and this curriculum will have the exact opposite impact as intended.

Instead, we have created this resource to be a tool to help you start the journey simply... and start with grace. You will find that the most effective path to wholeness in your health is not attempting some kind of quick sprint, but it is a consistent walk, where you incrementally "up" the pace as you are able.

Your Weekly Healthy and Free Schedule

- Small Group/Class Meeting: Watch the video session, dialogue, fellowship, and engage the activation exercise. Because the video sessions are shorter in length (8-15 minutes each), the goal is for participants to receive the information in smaller segments and discuss how to integrate it into everyday life.

▪ Monday–Friday Daily Readings: You will participate in the short, daily Healthy and Free devotional readings. These are designed to help reinforce the material you learned during the video session. (We also recommend reading the book as you go through the study, although you can go through the book at your preferred pace.)

These will be accompanied by *Healthy and Free* thoughts—simple summaries of the principle you have just ready about. Also, you will interact with the material and make it personal by going through the *Time to Reflect* questions.

Note: The purpose of the study guide readings and exercises is to help you reinforce the material you have been learning *and* interact with it. These activities should not take more than 15-20 minutes per day, at the maximum. The goal is to help you make information become activation that leads to personal transformation!

How Does This Work with the *Healthy and Free* Book?

You *can* go through the *Healthy and Free* curriculum without reading the book, although we highly recommend going through the study guide exercises *and* reading the book simultaneously.

Consider the *Healthy and Free* book your handbook. In the back, it contains many valuable resources that will help you along your journey (I'll refer to many of these during the video sessions).

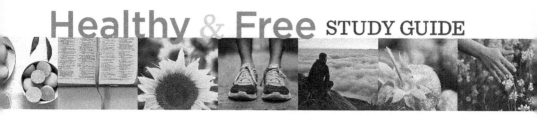

Session 1

Find Your Why

As you begin your own journey, I can't stress enough the importance of finding your "why." I promise you that it will help get you through so many challenges along the way. Maybe you want to become healthier because you'd like to be able to walk your daughter down the aisle at her wedding, or maybe you want your children to experience what it's like to have a parent who can play with them. Everyone has a different why. Don't wait until you are sick and have the doctor give you your why. Find your why with God now.

Session 1

Video Guide

Ten Steps to Beginning Your Health Journey

1. Find your _____

2. _____ with the Holy Spirit

3. Take _____ steps

4. Good health is not an _____

5. Have a vision for the _____ term

6. Recognize that this is a _____ change

7. Repent: change your _____

8. Always have _____

9. Give yourself _____

10. If you fail, get right back up and _____ going

11. Find your _____ journey

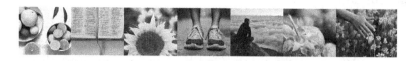

Weekly Health Practice

Find your "why" in order to sustain your journey toward health and wholeness.

Discussion Questions

1. What does it mean to find your why?

2. Discuss some ways that having a clearly identified why can help keep you motivated to stay on your health journey.

3. Share your personal stories—like mine—of your journey toward health.

4. What does it meant to give yourself grace during this lifestyle change? Why is grace so important in the process?

5. Discuss some "baby steps" you can take toward living a healthy and free lifestyle.

6. Why are baby steps so important (versus trying to make an instant and dramatic life overhaul)?

   Take a moment to break for the activation exercise.

Activation Exercise: Find Your Why

Today, you will *find your why*—and clearly identify you motivation for beginning and sustaining the journey toward health and wholeness.

Take some time to pray, reflect, and write down your *why*. Ask yourself:

- What is your motivation for getting healthy?

- What are the things God has put in your heart that He wants to do?

- Who are the people your life directly impacts?

- What are some things that you want to live to see?

- What do you envision yourself looking and feeling like 20 years from now?

You can work together in small groups if you feel comfortable discussing your *why* with each other. This might be a helpful practice to aid in coming up with different *whys*.

Resume Discussion Questions

7. Share your why (as you feel comfortable doing so). This exercise is designed to help you clarify a personal vision for pursuing a healthy and free lifestyle.

Weekly Exercises

Remember to engage your weekly activities in the study guide. While doing so, consider the following questions:

- What are some simple baby steps you can start taking toward living healthy?

- What are your health goals? (Writing these down and keeping them before you is always a helpful idea.)

One healthy meal won't solve all your problems, just like one unhealthy meal won't make you fat. It's a day-by-day, moment-by-moment walk with the Holy Spirit.

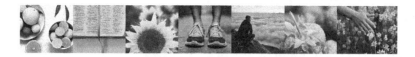

Find Your Why

*Do you not know that your bodies are temples of the
Holy Spirit, who is in you, whom you have received
from God? You are not your own; you were bought
at a price. Therefore honor God with your bodies.*
—1 CORINTHIANS 6:19-20 NIV

There are hundreds, if not thousands of messages, advertisements, and media-infused ideas all encouraging us to lose weight and become healthy. It seems that you cannot so much as drive two miles without being bombarded with billboards or bumper stickers that try to allure us with the promise of weight loss if we just follow their program. Why then are so many of us unhealthy if it seems that health programs are so readily accessible to us? The reason is because we haven't yet found our *why*. When you don't have a goal, saying yes to a cheeseburger and fries becomes too easy, because there isn't anything that will suffer from it. However, if we know and carry our why, we are then able to stand strong in the midst of temptation because we know what we want our end result to look like.

God designed us to be healthy and free. Health and wellness was His idea in the first place. Paul states in his letter to the church in Corinth that we were to honor God with our bodies because it is the place where the Holy Spirit makes His home within us. To put it in another perspective, imagine you were just informed that the President is going to be coming over to your house for dinner. How many of us would begin scrubbing and cleaning every nook and cranny we could find! We wouldn't dare invite the President into a home that is dirty and uncared for. The same should be true when it comes to our bodies because the Holy Spirit deserves the very best.

When we aren't healthy, we aren't feeling our best. When we aren't feeling our best, the people around us don't get to experience us in our full capacity. We are literally robbing the world of being able to experience what God created us to be. Let's commit to living our lives to our full potential. Let's commit to a life of health and freedom through Christ.

Healthy and Free Thought

Health was God's idea! We were never meant to live life in bondage to our bodies and food. We were created to be healthy and free!

Time to Reflect

1. What did Paul mean when he said that our bodies are the temple of the Holy Spirit?

_____

_____

_____

_____

_____

2. Have relationships in your life/dreams that you've had suffered because of your health?

_____

_____

_____

_____

_____

_____

3.   What is my why? Why am I going to be successful in this journey
     to health? Write your why in the space below.

_____

_____

_____

_____

_____

_____

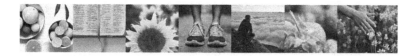

Let Go and Let God

*Remember not the former things, nor consider the
things of old. Behold, I am doing a new thing; now
it springs forth, do you not perceive it? I will make
a way in the wilderness and rivers in the desert.*
—Isaiah 43:18-19 ESV

We all have a story to tell. Many of our lives are rich with experiences of joy, happiness, loss, and heartaches. As we go through life, we knowingly and unknowingly make the decision to allow it to form us into who we are today. When we go through seasons of loss and sadness, we get to decide if we will allow these circumstances to make us stronger or make us bitter.

When it comes to our health, many of us have experienced difficulties or obstacles that may have discouraged or even halted our journey to wellness completely. Maybe it was a traumatic life event, a new job, a hurtful comment from a loved one, or just our own personal fear of succeeding.

Whatever it is, God is inviting you to let go of those experiences and take His hand as He leads you on this journey. God is inviting you in this journey to let go of the things that may have held you back in the past. Once you let go of the hurts and burdens, you can then more freely move into the life God created you to have…healthy and free.

Healthy and Free Thought

We were not created to live as slaves to our past! We have the ability to let go of the experiences and people who hurt us and to grab on to God.

Time to Reflect

1. What does the Bible say about holding on to bitterness and resentment?

_____

_____

_____

_____

_____

_____

_____

_____

2. How have you allowed your past to dictate your future?

_____

_____

_____

_____

_____

_____

_____

_____

3. What fears, challenges, or hurts do you need to let go of to truly walk in health and freedom? Ask the Holy Spirit to come and reveal these to you. He does not come with condemnation; rather, His conviction will empower you to start letting go of these hindrances to your wholeness and freedom!

_____

_____

_____

_____

_____

_____

Day 3

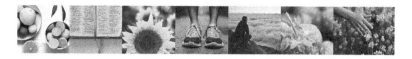

Taking the First Step

Therefore, if anyone is in Christ, the new creation
has come: The old has gone, the new is here!
—2 CORINTHIANS 5:17 NIV

Many of us come to a place in our lives where we realize that we have to make a change in one way or another. When it comes to getting healthy, it is easy to become overwhelmed when thinking of all the changes you may have to face. *"Drink more water! Exercise more! Rest! Go grocery shopping! Cook a healthy meal! Buy organic!"* Many times we allow ourselves to get so lost in the plethora of things that we may need to change that we instead choose to stay stagnant. Taking that first step on a lifelong journey can be intimidating, especially if you have a history of being unsuccessful with diets in the past. No one climbs an entire mountain successfully in one giant step. Instead, it's conquered one step at a time.

Ask yourself, "What step can I take for my health right now?" Maybe it's as simple as pouring yourself a tall glass of water as you read this or pausing to take three deep cleansing breaths. Whatever it is, that first step is going to make way for the next step, and the next, and the next. The hardest part of any journey is sometimes just getting started. Psalm 37:23 says, *"The Lord directs the steps of the godly. He delights in every detail of their lives."* God delights in *every* detail of our lives. Allow yourself to take your first step toward health today knowing that God is going to be taking great delight in it!

Healthy and Free Thought

God has promised to help guide our every step! We have been given the tools and ability to take our first steps into a healthy and free lifestyle!

Time to Reflect

1. What has prevented you from taking your first steps into health and wellness?

_____

_____

_____

_____

_____

_____

_____

2. What are some practical steps that you can take today that will help start you on this journey?

_____

_____

_____

_____

_____

_____

3. How will remembering your *why* help you take those first steps?

_____

_____

_____

_____

_____

_____

_____

_____

Day 4

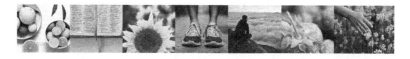

Lean on the Holy Spirit

*For I hold you by your right hand —I, the
Lord your God. And I say to you, "Don't
be afraid. I am here to help you."*
—Isaiah 41:13

Have you ever been to a new city or country and found yourself overwhelmed with having to navigate your way through a new and unfamiliar place? Many times we have to rely on maps, a tour guide, or a friendly city-dweller to help guide us to where we need to be. Well, I'd like to invite you to think of the Holy Spirit as your "go-to" tour guide on this journey! As we read yesterday in Psalm 37, the Lord loves to be involved with every detail of our lives, and this includes our health. Health was God's idea in the first place. He knows what steps you need to take in order to get healthy better than anyone else and wants to help guide you!

In *Healthy and Free,* I tell the story of when I first began my health journey. I knew that the Lord had told me to get healthy, but I had no idea where to start. I prayed and asked the Holy Spirit and very clearly heard Him say to cut out refined sugar. The Lord was faithful to direct my steps the entire way, as He will be with you. If you find yourself lost and overwhelmed, just remember that sometimes we all need to stop and ask for directions.

Healthy and Free Thought

This journey is an adventure with the Holy Spirit! You don't need to feel overwhelmed or lost because you have the Him to help show you the way.

Time to Reflect

1. Ask the Holy Spirit what He thinks about this journey you are on. What did you hear Him say?

_____

_____

_____

_____

_____

_____

_____

2. What are some of the first steps you feel the Holy Spirit is leading you to take?

_____

_____

_____

_____

_____

_____

_____

3. How will leaning on the Holy Spirit during this journey help you be more successful than other times you may have tried to get healthy?

_____

_____

_____

_____

_____

_____

_____

_____

Day 5

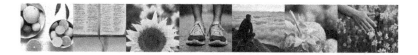

You Are Powerful!

For I can do everything through
Christ, who gives me strength.
—Philippians 4:13

We live in a culture where we measure our worth based on our success. There are hundreds of wide-ranging diets out there that all try to entice us to find our value and a "better life" through its program. Unfortunately, 95 percent of people who diet oftentimes fail. It leaves them feeling powerless and causes an increase in low self-esteem. If you have found yourself in that 95 percent at one time or another, today is the day to leave those old mindsets of failure behind you and to embrace the truth of who God says you are—powerful!

God created health, but He did not create diets. We were never meant to live in a vicious cycle that exhausts every part of our being. We were created from a powerful DNA source, our Heavenly Father, and we have been given the tools to live powerfully. Second Timothy 1:7 says, *"God has not given us a spirit of fear, but of power and of love and of a sound mind"* (NKJV). No longer do we have to live in fear of failure, rejection, or disappointment! We have been freely given the spirit of power, love, and peace from our Heavenly Father. Today I want to invite you to let go of the lie that you are powerless and embrace the truth that you are powerful.

Healthy and Free Thought

God has given you the tools to be powerful in every situation in your life. You were made to be powerful and victorious!

Time to Reflect

1. How has the lie that you are powerless held you back in the past?

    _____

    _____

    _____

    _____

    _____

    _____

    _____

    _____

2. How will grabbing hold of the truth that you are powerful (in Christ, through the empowerment of the Holy Spirit) help your journey in health?

    _____

    _____

    _____

    _____

    _____

    _____

    _____

3. What are some practical tools you can use when you feel the powerless lie try to creep back in?

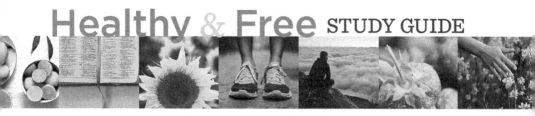

Session 2

The Secret Power
of Soul Health

There is something powerful about loving God, being loved by Him, loving yourself, and then being able to give that same love to those around you that brings incredible health and life to our lives, and it all starts in our minds.

Session 2

Video Guide

Soul: The essential life of man; it is looking earthward.

Keys to Change Your Thinking

1. We need to _____ ourselves.

2. Give yourself _____.

3. _____ to yourself.

4. _____ yourself.

5. Believe what God _____ about you.

6. _____ at the negative thoughts.

7. Start out your day thinking _____ thoughts.

8. Give the Holy Spirit permission to _____ your mind.

9. Make _____.

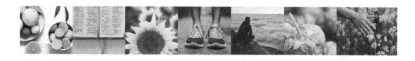

Weekly Health Practice

Create a healthy thought life: If you want to change your life, start changing the way you think!

Discussion Questions

1. What is the difference between the spirit and soul?

2. How are the soul and mind as one?

3. How can negative thoughts cause poor soul health?

4. How does the process of repentance impact your thought life?

5. Based on Matthew 22:37-40, why do you think it's so important to love yourself and how does this contribute to soul health?

6. How can laughing change the way you think? Impact your thought life? Change your perspective on circumstances you are dealing with?

7. How can laughing actually strip lies of their power over your thinking?

8. Explain how making declarations can change the way you think. Why is it important for truth to be on your lips? How does hearing your mouth say truth change the way you think?

Activation Exercise: Laugh at the Lies...and Throw Them Away

Today, you will *laugh at the lies*—and then throw them in the garbage. You will need paper and pencils/pens.

Identify the Lies

Take some time to pray, reflect, and write down some of the most common lies that you deal with. (Don't write your name on the paper, because it will ultimately end up in the trash.)

Laugh at the Lies

If you feel lead by the Holy Spirit, you can look at the lies you have believed and laugh at them. This will take an act of willpower, because these lies have been no laughing matter in the past. In fact, they have been tormenting for so many people. Laughing at them is one key way of breaking agreement with lies.

By laughing, you are denying lies their power over your life.

Throw the Lies in the Trash

After laughing at the lies, wad/rip up the paper and throw it into a garbage bin (as a prophetic act).

Weekly Exercises

Engage your weekly activities in the study guide. While doing so, consider the following questions:

- What are some reoccurring lies the enemy continues to bombard your mind with? (Be aware of these, because they will most likely come back and you need to be ready to reject them.)

- Remember the prophetic act you made by tearing up the lies and throwing them into the trash; this must be your response any time these lies come back.

- Over the week, write down the truth of what God says about you (what God says about you versus what the lie said).

You can find more information about this process in Chapter 2 of the *Healthy and Free* book.

Having a healthy mind is just as important as having a healthy body. In fact, when we have good thoughts about ourselves, it actually causes our whole being to respond in a positive way.

Day 6

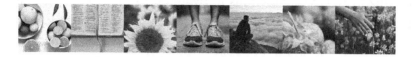

Mind Health

Fix your thoughts on what is true, and honorable, and right, and pure, and lovely, and admirable. Think about things that are excellent and worthy of praise.
—PHILIPPIANS 4:8

Many times when people think of getting healthy, they see rows of weights, treadmills, and kitchens stocked with apples and kale galore. While working out and eating healthy are a few keys to help make our bodies well, we often forget about another very important part of a healthy lifestyle—our minds.

I want to start off by encouraging you to not carelessly skip through the process of getting your soul healthy. It is easy to focus on the more natural progressions of health like food and exercise, but I can promise you that the benefits that you will reap from exercising your mind will only help accelerate your success in the long run.

We are triune beings made of a body, soul, and spirit. Our souls (also known as our minds) have the power to either help or work against our journeys to health. We have the ability to talk our bodies into either being healthy or unhealthy, and it all comes from the power of our thoughts. Having a healthy body will almost happen naturally when we have a healthy mind.

The apostle Paul instructs us to "fix our minds on things above" (see Col. 3:2) meaning to align our thoughts with Heaven. This can be a fairly difficult thing to do in the midst of the hustle and bustle of our daily lives. Getting the kids ready and off to school, errands, jobs, bills, cleaning, getting dinners ready, etc. can all cause us to lose focus and let our frustrations take precedence in our minds. However, the act of exercising our minds and allowing ourselves to see Heaven's point of view over our circumstances will help not only shift our perspective but possibly the outcome of our lives as well.

Healthy and Free Thought

It is impossible to have a fully healthy body without a healthy mind. Aligning our thoughts with Heaven will be the catapult that will accelerate us on this journey.

Time to Reflect

1. Review Colossians 3:2. What did Paul mean when he said to fix our minds on things above, and how does that play into our journey to wellness?

_____

_____

_____

_____

_____

_____

2. Being completely honest with yourself, how healthy is your mind if you had to rate it? (Are the majority of your thoughts positive or negative?)

_____

_____

_____

_____

_____

_____

_____

3. How is having a healthy mind important to our bodies/physical
    health?

_____

_____

_____

_____

_____

_____

_____

Day 7

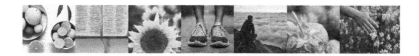

Repent and Change
Your Mind

*I cannot afford to have a thought in
my head that is not in His.*
—BILL JOHNSON

This week, we discussed and explored the idea of loving who you are. For some of us, this topic may have stirred up old mindsets or unhealthy thought patterns that we have been accustomed to living with. A crucial part of keeping your soul healthy is taking those thoughts captive and changing them to come in line with God's.

Bill Johnson often says, "I cannot afford to have a thought in my head that is not in His." The first step that comes with renewing your mind is repentance. There is something powerful behind repenting for believing the lies that the enemy has tried to destroy our very beings with and not believing what God has to say about us.

Repentance means to "turn around." When we turn our thoughts away from the negative and destructive patterns of thinking, we have to intentionally turn our mind around, shifting our thinking toward thoughts that bring life and joy. Paul instructs us in Colossians to "also rid yourselves of all such things as these: anger, rage, malice, slander, and filthy language from your lips" (see Col. 3:8). Many times we read this verse assuming that he was referring to our speech and actions toward others; however, I'd like to propose to you that it is also applicable in how we speak and act toward *ourselves*.

As with any new habit, it may seem uncomfortable and unending at first. We have on average 30,000 thoughts a day, so trying to catch every one can be overwhelming! But you will notice that over time, the negative thoughts will begin to shift on their own. It will no longer be hard work to try and change your mind, Because you'll have a foundation that is focused on how God sees you. Any thought that tries to convince you of a reality that is contrary to what God says about you will be immediately identified and rejected for what it is—a lie!

Healthy and Free Thought

Having a thought about ourselves that is not in alignment with God's thoughts is a direct violation of who God created us to be.

Time to Reflect

1. If someone were to overhear the way you talked to yourself, what would they have to say?

_____

_____

_____

_____

_____

_____

_____

2. Repent and take a moment to ask the Lord what He has to say about you. What was His response? If you need some help getting started, I encourage you to read Psalm 139.

_____

_____

_____

_____

_____

_____

_____

3. How will you be sure to steward the words that God has to say about you? List some practical ways that you can stay mindful of God's thoughts toward you.

_____

_____

_____

_____

_____

_____

_____

_____

Day 8

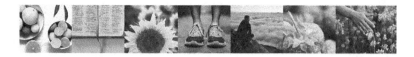

Learning to Love Ourselves

*Anyone who knows who God made them to
be will never try to be someone else.*
—BILL JOHNSON

Loving ourselves is perhaps one of the most vital keys to successfully becoming healthy because health is a form of self-love. Many of us come from all different backgrounds in life and carry different experiences that helped shape how we see ourselves. Some may have come from abusive homes where value and love weren't displayed. Others may have been abandoned, bullied at school, emotionally abused, and the list goes on. Many times when this happens, the enemy uses it to try to make us lessen our own value and self-love. Whatever your situation was, I want to invite you to fall in love with yourself again.

Falling in love with yourself is an art. Many people expect to be able to say one prayer or one declaration and be set free from self-hate. Even though that is a possibility, many times it's an ongoing process. Oftentimes, we do not fall in love with another person just after one coffee meet-up or date, but we fall in love as we pursue and get to know the other person on a more intimate level.

Today, I want to encourage you to begin to pursue yourself. Take yourself out to coffee, write a love letter to yourself, and look at yourself in the mirror as if you're the most beautiful person you have ever laid eyes on. Whatever loving yourself looks like to you, do it. Make yourself a priority.

If we could only grasp the depth of God's love for us, we wouldn't dare do anything to violate the one thing He gave His life to save—*ourselves*. Remember, you can only love to the degree that you are loved.

Today, let's love the very thing Jesus died to save.

Healthy and Free Thought

Loving ourselves is the key to making a lasting change in our lives. Without self-love, we cannot be successful at pursuing a healthy lifestyle because health is a side effect of self-love.

Time to Reflect

Before doing the reflection questions, today I want you to do something kind for yourself. Then, come back to the study and answer the questions.

1. What did you do as an act of loving yourself and how did you feel after?

_____

_____

_____

_____

_____

_____

_____

_____

_____

_____

2.   What are three things you love about yourself and why?

_____

_____

_____

_____

_____

_____

_____

_____

_____

_____

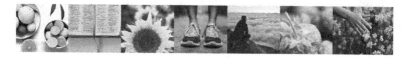

The Power of Laughter

A joyful heart is good medicine, but a
crushed spirit dries up the bones.
—Proverbs 17:22 ESV

There is nothing quite like a good laugh. Now I don't mean an almost silent "hmm" after someone tells a mediocre joke, but the kind that makes you bend over, abs hurting, and tears streaming down your face type of laughter. Once you've calmed down and can finally catch your breath, it's almost as if you feel refreshed and life's problems don't seem to have the same sense of urgency that they did just minutes prior. Of course, there is a scientific reason for that being that laughter produces endorphins, also known as the "happy hormone." But beyond that, I believe that it also helps heal and strengthen us on a spiritual level.

Joy is such a vital part of the gospel. Hebrews 12:2 says, *"Because of the joy awaiting him, he endured the cross, disregarding its shame."* Jesus had the power and ability to move past any shame that may have tried to rear its ugly head at Him and look forward with great expectation because He knew that joy was just around the corner.

All throughout Scripture, we see joy as a theme. Proverbs 15:15 says, *"The cheerful of heart has a continual feast"* (ESV). Joy is one of Heaven's greatest weapons against the enemy because it gives us the ability to persevere despite our surroundings. Joy fuels our hope and releases breakthrough in times of suffering.

If you feel that you've lost your joy, today is your day to reignite that flame. Joy to the believer should be as natural as breathing. I want to invite you to pray the prayer below if you feel you need help finding your joy again.

> *Father, I ask that You forgive me for losing my joy. I thank You that joy is what You promised to every believer and that it is readily available for me today. I pray that You fill my heart with joy and reveal to me any area of my life where joy is needed to release healing. I thank You, Jesus, for enduring the cross for me and for releasing supernatural joy to those You love.*

Healthy and Free Thought

Joy is the key to experiencing and persevering for breakthrough in our lives! Joy releases supernatural ability to do things we may not have been able to do otherwise.

Time to Reflect

1. How will incorporating joy into your life help accelerate you on the journey toward health and wholeness?

_____

_____

_____

_____

_____

_____

2. What are some practical tools you can implement to make sure you steward joy in your life?

_____

_____

_____

_____

_____

_____

_____

3. Are there any areas of your life where joy has been absent? What does the Holy Spirit say about these areas?

_____

_____

_____

_____

_____

_____

_____

Day 10

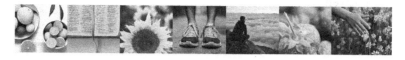

The Power of Declarations

The tongue has the power of life and death,
and those who love it will eat its fruit.
—Proverbs 18:21 NIV

The power of life and death are in the tongue. That's a pretty bold statement when you stop to think about it. In a culture where words are thrown out more carelessly than one's trash, that can be a pretty scary thought. On the flip side, words can also be used to bring life to the very thing they once tried to destroy.

Job 22:28 states that *"you will also decree a thing, and it will be established for you; and light will shine on your ways"* (NASB). When we speak, we are creating a momentum for change in the spiritual realm that eventually will take its place in the physical realm. When it comes to health, many people have spoken negative words against themselves by saying things like, "I cannot lose weight," or "I always fail," or even "I'll probably always be fat!" As it turns out, that becomes their personal truth because they have spoken that into existence. Henry Ford said it best when he said, "Whether you think you can or you can't, you're right."

On the other hand, when we speak words that are aligned with Heaven, God actually partners with us and breathes life on those words. As if that isn't powerful enough, the more we speak those declarations out, the more our mind begins to transform and renew itself with the truth of Heaven.

Healthy and Free Thought

We get to choose whether our words will make or break our lives. Godly declarations carry a supernatural ability to transform our minds, lives, and even bodies.

Time to Reflect

1. Take a moment to ask the Holy Spirit if you have knowingly or unknowingly spoken any negative words against yourself and your journey toward health. What did He show you?

_____

_____

_____

_____

_____

_____

2. What are three declarations you can choose to speak over yourself daily?

_____

_____

_____

_____

_____

_____

3. How will changing your speech help improve not only your health journey, but also your overall quality of life?

_____

_____

_____

_____

_____

_____

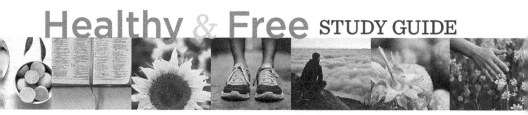

Session 3

The Body, Soul, and Spirit Connection

Just as the Father, Son, and the Holy Spirit are a triune God, we are also created as a triune being. We are body, soul, and spirit. The beauty and mystery of the Godhead is that there is no separation between the three. They are different and yet the same. Because we are made in His image, the same is true for us. There is no separation between our bodies, souls, and spirits. We have to see ourselves as this whole being and appreciate how God made us without elevating one part over another.

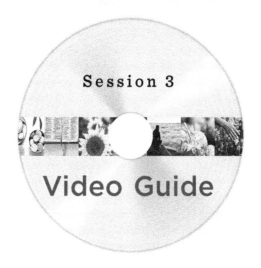

Session 3

Video Guide

1. It is our _____ to take care of God's temple—our bodies.

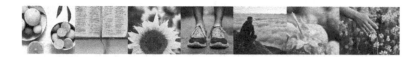

Weekly Health Practice

Recognize the connection: Your body, soul, and spirit function together and the health in one realm directly impacts the health in another.

Discussion Questions

1. How have your understood the body-soul-spirit connection in the past?

2. How can health in one area directly impact another?

3. Discuss the concept of being the temple of the Holy Spirit from 1 Corinthians 6:19. What are the implications of our bodies being the actual temple of God on earth? Discuss what this means.

4. How should really understanding this truth—that we are God's temple—impact the way we approach our health?

5. What are some ways we can take care of God's temple?

6. When you understand how intricately God designed you, how does this change the way you view your life? Your purpose?

7. How does it change the way you view your body when you understand that the Spirit of God chose to live inside of you?

Activation Exercise: If Your Body Is the Temple of God...

Oftentimes, we throw around phrases and statements so frequently that we stop reflecting on their deeper meaning. This tends to be the case with what Paul wrote about our bodies being the temple of the Holy Spirit.

Today, you will take time to meditate and reflect on what the following Scriptures *really mean* and how their truth should impact the way you approach your life—body, soul, and spirit.

Meditate on the Word (5-10 minutes)

Take the following passages of Scripture and reflectively meditate on the truth they communicate.

> *Or do you not know that your body is the temple of the Holy Spirit who is in you, whom you have from God, and you are not your own? For you were bought at a price; therefore glorify God in your body and in your spirit, which are God's* (1 Corinthians 6:19-20 NKJV)

> *You are Christ's body—that's who you are!* (1 Corinthians 12:27 MSG)

Journal (10 minutes)

Write down *what* it means for your body to be a temple of the Holy Spirit. If God lives inside of you, how then should you treat your body?

_____

_____

_____

_____

_____

_____

_____

_____

_____

_____

_____

_____

_____

_____

_____

Write down *what* it means for you to be part of the body of Christ—that Jesus has chosen people to make up His body on the earth.

_____

_____

_____

_____

_____

_____

_____

_____

_____

_____

_____

_____

_____

_____

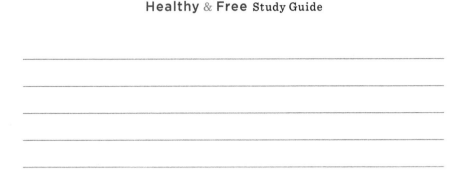

_____

_____

_____

_____

_____

Engage

Share your meditations and reflections on what it means for us to be 1) the temple of the Holy Spirit and 2) the body of Christ. How should this impact the way we live? Eat? Exercise? What we watch? What we give our time to? This is not a call to be religious, focusing on "dos" and "donts." Instead, it's about stewarding the Presence of the Holy Spirit who lives inside of us.

Weekly Exercises

Engage your weekly activities in the study guide. While doing so, meditate on the following passages of Scripture:

- 1 Corinthians 6:19-20

- 1 Corinthians 3:16-17

- Romans 12:1-2

- Ephesians 2:21

You can find more information about this process in Chapter 3 of the *Healthy and Free* book.

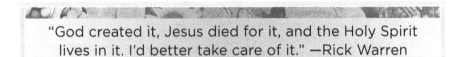

"God created it, Jesus died for it, and the Holy Spirit lives in it. I'd better take care of it." —Rick Warren

Day 11

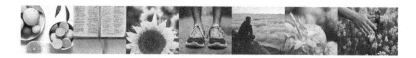

God's Art

You made all the delicate, inner parts of my body
and knit me together in my mother's womb.
—Psalm 139:13

Since the beginning of time, God has been an artist. He painted the detailed colors and shadows in the sky as the sun rises and sets. He formed the depths of the oceans and crafted the highest of mountains. His ability to create and design is beyond our comprehension as science still continues to discover intricate details of all He has breathed His life on. Yet despite the beauty of a sunset and the mystery of a vast forest, His finest, most impressive work of art is us. Our bodies are of great importance to God.

Another way to think about this is to imagine that God owned a garden. Its roses were always in full bloom and you could smell them the moment you stepped foot on its green grass. The trees grew tall and strong and every plant had been properly trimmed and pruned. Now imagine He decided to hand over His gardening tools and put you in charge of His garden. I can only imagine that every one of us would be careful and intentional to not destroy a single rose, tree, or plant and would work diligently to keep it in prime condition. It may even require a bit of sacrifice from our end—which may not be easy in the moment—but knowing His satisfaction in seeing us care about the very thing He entrusted to us would be worth it.

Now imagine that the garden in the picture I just painted for you represents your body. The detail and care That went into His intricate design when He created us far exceeds any of His other wonders in creation. In the church, we in generally have focused on keeping our spirits healthy, but have often completely neglected keeping our bodies healthy.

As you go through this week's study, I want you to remind yourself that you've been entrusted with the very thing that Jesus came to save. You've been entrusted to care for and steward your body—the craftsmanship of God and the temple of the Holy Spirit!

Healthy and Free Thought

> Our bodies are God's greatest work of art. Caring for our physical health is a great honor for us as believers, as it pleases the heart of God to see us value the very thing He gave to us.

Time to Reflect

1. Sit and close your eyes for a moment. Imagine that your body represents a garden. When you are walking through this garden, what do you notice? Is it clean and well-kept? Has it been deserted?

_____

_____

_____

_____

_____

_____

_____

2.   In what ways could you improve the condition of your garden? List these below.

_____

_____

_____

_____

_____

_____

_____

_____

_____

_____

_____

_____

_____

_____

_____

_____

_____

Even if you end up writing a longer list, remember, don't allow that to overwhelm you! The journey toward health and wholeness is one baby step at a time.

Day 12

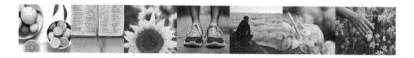

Experiencing the Triune Connection

Hope deferred makes the heart sick, but
a dream fulfilled is a tree of life.
—PROVERBS 13:12

Emotions play a vital part in our lives. Our lives are full of them ranging from joy to heartache, from love to depression. Did you know that emotions actually not only affect our spirits and hearts, but also our bodies? There have been many studies that show when emotions are experienced they get stored in our bodies. A study done at Harvard University showed that people who had experienced traumatic or anxiety-ridden events in their lives later go on to have stomach problems because the brain and digestive system are intricately connected.[1] Fascinating! On the other hand, it's also been proven that laughter (joy) can actually bring healing and rid the body of sickness as well.[2] It's a beautiful example of how God created us as triune beings.

Today, we are going to explore some emotions that you may have experienced in the past and break off any residue that they may have left behind in your body. Take a moment to close your eyes and ask the Holy Spirit to bring to your mind a time when a negative emotion may have tried to find its home in your body. After the Lord shows you, allow yourself to go back to that place and take note of any emotions or thoughts you may have had. I want you to use this next page to journal some of your thoughts.

- What happened?

- What is my body feeling? Sadness? Anxiety?

- Where in my body am I feeling these emotions?

- What thoughts am I having?

Now, I want you to ask the Holy Spirit to speak the truth to you over that situation.

- What does God have to say about the moment/experience He is revealing to you?

- As you take His words to heart, how does your body begin to feel? Does it relax? Do you feel peace? Allow yourself to really feel what may be changing in your body.

Now, I want you to lay hands over the area of your body that may have been affected by this and pray this prayer:

Father, I break agreement with (negative emotion you felt) and I declare that my body is whole and healed. I speak peace over my body and I give my body permission to fully live and operate just as God intended it to. I thank You, Father, that You see every part of me and Your will is to see me healed and whole. I declare my wholeness in Your name.

You may need to repeat this process a few times if you feel it necessary. Remember, this is a journey. As the Lord continues to reveal to you memories or experiences, allow yourself to go through the process in order for Him to bring you complete healing.

Healthy and Free Thought

Because our being—spirit, soul, and body—is connected, emotions and experiences can become stored in our body. It is important to let go of those negative emotions in order for our bodies to experience full healing.

Time to Reflect

1. Describe the experience as you allowed yourself to feel any negative emotions that may have been stored in your body.

---

2. Why is it important to be aware of your emotions and their impact on your body?

Note

1. Anthony L. Komaroff, "The Gut-brain Connection," Harvard Health, March 27, 2012, http://www.health.harvard.edu/healthbeat/the-gut-brain-connection.

2. Health, "How Happiness Affects Your Health," ABC News, May 27, 2013, http://abcnews.go.com/blogs/health/2013/03/27/how-happiness-affects-your-health/.

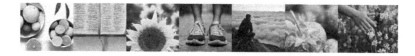

The World Needs Healthy Christians

I want to live to see the day that churches are a place for wellness that the world goes to and looks to as the source.
—JORDAN RUBIN

Most of us are familiar with the apostle Paul. He is perhaps most known for his travels and successful promotion of the gospel. Now, we have no way of knowing what Paul looked like, what he weighed, or what his diet consisted of. However, it may be safe to say that perhaps Paul understood the importance of taking care of his physical body. He traveled thousands upon thousands of miles in his lifetime and he would have had to be healthy to do so, especially in a time when airplanes, cars, and buses did not exist. While some of us may not dream of traveling the world to preach, we have been commissioned to spread the Gospel in whatever sphere of influence we have been called to. We can never minister to our neighbors down the street if we are too tired to get off the couch.

The world needs healthy Christians. The Holy Spirit spoke to me and said that He wants me around for the long haul. I believe this is His message for you too! While our individual callings may look different, the world needs what we have to offer. This is a perfect explanation as to why our bodies, souls, and spirits all are of great importance. We need our bodies to deliver the message that our spirits have received that our minds help us process and communicate effectively!

Healthy and Free Thought

The world needs what we carry through Christ. Without mind, body, and spirit health, we cannot live and promote the gospel to our fullest potential.

Time to Reflect

1. How is having a healthy body, soul, and spirit important to your destiny as a believer?

_____

_____

_____

_____

_____

_____

_____

2. How will being healthy directly impact the call on your life?

_____

_____

_____

_____

_____

_____

3. In what ways could being healthy change the world around you?

_____

_____

_____

_____

_____

_____

_____

Day 14

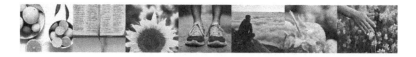

Experiencing God in Total Health

*Dear friend, I pray that you may enjoy good
health and that all may go well with you,
even as your soul is getting along well.*
—3 John 1:2 NIV

The Bible tells us that we were created in the image of God. While that may have a few different meanings, it also refers to the fact that we are a triune being. Being a triune being, we were meant to experience God through our body, soul, and spirit in His fullness. Many times we limit our encounters with God to just our spirits, but John 10:10 says that Jesus came that we may have life and life to the full! That means we were created to be fulfilled in every aspect—including our body, soul, and spirit.

As we discussed yesterday, the world needs healthy Christians. Today, I'd like to propose to you the idea that God needs healthy Christians as well. Have you ever had a friend or family member who was sick? Seeing them suffer can be heavy on our hearts and we long for the day when they are well again. We aren't able to experience relationship with that person to the full extent that we would if they were well. We begin to miss the way they used to be before sickness overtook them. The same is true in our relationship with God. He desires to see His children well because that's when He truly sees and gets the best of us. Only when we are able to offer our best is He able to fully commune with us.

Healthy and Free Thought

God deserves our very best. When we are sick and unhealthy, we rob Him from experiencing us at our fullest potential.

Time to Reflect

1. What would it look like to live to your fullest potential in body, soul, and spirit?

_____

_____

_____

_____

_____

_____

2. How can being healthy actually change our relationship with God?

_____

_____

_____

_____

_____

_____

_____

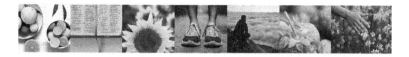

Visualize Your Why

Agree with God, and be at peace;
thereby good will come to you.
—Job 22:21 ESV

By now, you have worked through some aspects of spirit and soul health as well as having a greater understanding for how the body, soul, and spirit all work together. As you continue to steward your health in these areas, you will begin to see noticeable changes in yourself.

You may notice that your confidence has been strengthened or that you're beginning to not only *like* yourself, but also *love* yourself. When you are operating to your fullest potential in all three areas of your being, you are then able to fully experience the life God intended you to have.

Today, I want to take you on a journey. I want to give you permission dream of the life you have ahead of you. In life, it is vital that you have a vision for yourself whether it's for your career, fitness, or relationships. Having vision is what will help push you forward when you feel like giving up. In short, you are going to visualize your *why*.

Take a moment and imagine your ideal life 10 years from now. You can take as long as you need to on this exercise. There is only one rule. You have to be unafraid to dream…and dream big! As you visualize what you want your life to look like in 10 years, ask yourself these questions:

- What does your dream life look like?

- What does your body look like?

- Does it feel healthy and strong?

- Picture the people in your life whom you love—like family and friends. How has becoming healthy affected those relationships?

- Have they been motivated by your journey to become healthy themselves?

- Imagine how you move about your day in your healthy body. How does it feel different from the body you had before?

- Imagine how your confidence and self-esteem feel.

- How has your relationship with God changed since your journey began?

Whenever you feel like you may have lost vision for yourself, you can always come back to today's study and walk yourself through visualizing your why.

Healthy and Free Thought

God intended us to be fully alive and fully healthy in body, soul, and spirit! As we continue to grow in every aspect of our being, God continues to partner with us to take us even further in our journey.

Time to Reflect

1. Why is having vision for your life helpful to you being successful on your journey?

_____

_____

_____

_____

_____

2.   Take time to ask the Holy Spirit what He thinks about the
     dreams you have for yourself. What did He have to say?

_____

_____

_____

_____

_____

_____

_____

_____

_____

_____

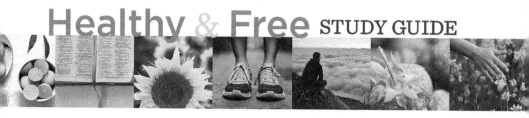

Session 4

The Power of Sleep and Water

When I am asked what I believe is the most important healthy life practice, I always say drinking water. This is one practice that will instantly help you move toward living the *Healthy and Free* lifestyle.

In addition, quality rest is absolutely essential to sustaining your health journey. Sleep is the foundation for good health because without it, the body simply cannot reap the benefits of a healthy lifestyle. Sleeping will help you mentally and emotionally, too. Don't be afraid to allow yourself to relax and get a good amount of sleep. Whatever you have on your to-do list will still be there tomorrow when you get up. Only then you'll be well rested and in a better place spiritually, mentally, and physically to accomplish all that you need to get done.

Session 4

Video Guide

Facts about H$_2$0

1. Your body is made up of at least _____ percent water.

2. If you are thirsty, you are starting
    to _____.

3. Water _____ your body.

4. Water will _____ and hydrate your
    body.

Some Solutions for Sleeping Disorders

1. Sit outside in the _____ for 10 minutes.

2. Take _____ for relaxation and digestion.

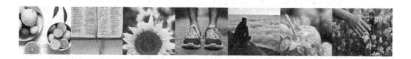

Weekly Health Practice

Rest and hydrate: Drinking water and practicing good sleep habits are vital to living healthy and free.

Discussion Questions

1. Why do you think it's so important to drink lots of water?

2. What do people often drink instead of water? (How can these substitutes be damaging?)

3. Discuss why you think many people neglect drinking water.

4. What do you currently do when you feel thirsty? What should you be doing?

5. How has our culture become sleep deprived? List and discuss some of the things that prevent people from sleeping and getting good rest.

6. Share about your journey into rest. If you have overcome a sleep disorder, share your story (if you feel comfortable doing so) and, specifically, describe what steps were helpful in overcoming the disorder.

Activation Exercise: Two Steps toward Health and Wholeness

Today, we are going to identify two steps we can take toward greater health and wholeness: One step in hydration and one step in rest. *That's it!*

Remember to make the steps "baby steps." In other words, you might not want to do something drastic like completely quitting drinking soda and switching to all water, or immediately changing your sleep hours to 10 p.m. until 6 a.m. We recommend you *begin a journey* in both areas.

Here is what we will do:

1. Either as a group/class or smaller groups, openly discuss different steps that could be great places to start for drinking more water and getting better rest.

2. Write down the different suggestions and evaluate what might work best for your personal journeys.

Weekly Exercises

Engage your weekly activities in the study guide. While doing so, stick with practicing your two steps—one for drinking water and one for getting better rest. *Do not* add any other steps to the process yet. Right now, the most important thing is getting started! Once momentum picks up and you feel comfortable with your two new steps as a routine, you can identify the next necessary steps to take.

You can find more information about this process in Chapter 4 of the *Healthy and Free* book.

Don't be afraid to allow yourself to relax and get a good amount of sleep.

Day 16

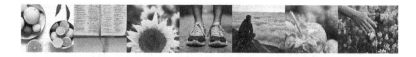

Water

But whoever drinks of the water that I will
give him will never be thirsty again. The water
that I will give him will become in him a
spring of water welling up to eternal life.
—John 4:14 ESV

Throughout the gospels, we often hear Jesus refer to the life He brings as "living water." He promises that those who believe in Him will "never be thirsty again." Jesus used this metaphor to paint a picture of how the spirit suffers without the water of the spirit just as the body suffers without natural water.

Illustrating the Gospel using water is powerful because it shows the vast importance that water has to our bodies. Just like the Gospel, water brings healing and health as well as helps restore our bodies back to the way God intended them to be. Without water, our bodies are unable to function just as our spirits are unable to function without our "living water." The human body can survive weeks without food, but only three to five days without drinking water before it begins to shut down.

Many of us are dehydrated and have absolutely no idea. So, today's challenge is to simply drink more water. A good rule of thumb when figuring out how much water to drink is to drink half of your body weight in ounces. If that sounds too extreme for you, simply count how many glasses of water you normally drink in a day and add two extra glasses to that. Once your body begins to be properly hydrated, you will be amazed at how much better your body will feel.

Healthy and Free Thought

Water is of such importance to our bodies that Jesus compared the life He brought to us as "living water." We need water to survive both in the natural and spiritual.

Time to Reflect

1. Why is it important to make proper hydration a part of your daily life?

_____

_____

_____

_____

_____

_____

2. How does Jesus comparing the Gospel to water show the importance that water has in our lives?

_____

_____

_____

_____

_____

_____

_____

3. What practical steps can you implement to make sure you are receiving good water throughout your day?

_____

_____

_____

_____

_____

_____

_____

_____

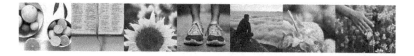

Quality Versus Quantity

Water is the driving force of all nature.
—Leonardo da Vinci

As with anything we partake of in life, quality far outweighs quantity. The same is true when it comes to the water we drink. In today's world, most of our tap water contains numerous chemicals and additives that may only cause more problems down the line when ingested. One may be drinking their daily needed intake of water, but if the water is packed with toxins, it may have the opposite effect on the body than desired. This is why investing in a water purifier would have long-term health benefits to you.

Another important key to factor in is to make it a point to alkalize your body. An alkalized body is a disease-free body. Now don't allow the word *alkalize* to intimidate you. Alkalizing your body can be as simple as squeezing half a lemon or lime into your water! This is going to bring health and happiness to your entire body, primarily your digestive system.

Today's challenge is short and sweet. Alkalize your body! Pour yourself a tall glass of water, add some lemon or lime and drink up! This is a good habit to create especially first thing in the morning. After a few days, you will feel a noticeable difference in your body's overall performance.

Healthy and Free Thought

Quality of water far outweighs the quantity of water! Finding good, pure water and alkalizing your body will bring lasting health and wellness and is another way you can be sure to steward the body God gave you.

Time to Reflect

1. What are some practical steps you can take to make sure you are giving your body pure, clean water on a daily basis?

_____

_____

_____

_____

_____

_____

2. How is the simple act of adding lemon to your water beneficial to you?

_____

_____

_____

_____

_____

_____

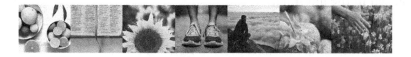

The Power of Sleep

For God gives rest to his loved ones.
—Psalm 127:2

Anyone who has missed out on a good night's sleep knows that sleep is serious business! Without it, it is nearly impossible to make it throughout our day without at least one minor breakdown. Psalm 127:2 states that the Lord "grants sleep to those he loves" (NIV). That's a powerful statement! Sleep is of great importance when pursuing a life of health and wellness and yet is perhaps one of the most overlooked aspects as well.

Sleep was God's idea from the beginning. If He intended for us to live off of caffeine and three hours of sleep, He would have created our bodies to be able to do so. However, He created our bodies to need rest. Sleep is what helps restore and protect our bodies against the stress of our day-to-day lives. Without it, healthy foods and exercise can only go so far.

Many of us live busy lives. We have to balance kids, homework, schoolwork, housework, cooking, cleaning, a job, family, friends, exercise, etc.! It is easy to put sleep at the bottom of our to-do list. Today's challenge is going to be a little different from our previous studies. I want you right now to set a time in which you will go to bed tonight and make a promise to yourself that no matter how many dishes need to be done and no matter how intriguing that TV show is, you are going to go to bed at this time. I can almost guarantee that you'll thank yourself in the morning.

Healthy and Free Thought

Sleep is a key component to achieving and maintaining a healthy lifestyle. Without proper rest, all our other efforts are almost obsolete if the body is not given enough rest to reap the benefits.

Time to Reflect

1. What thoughts/feelings come to mind when you are asked to commit to putting everything on your to-do list aside to make sure you get to bed at a proper time?

_____

_____

_____

_____

_____

2. How will making sleep a priority positively affect not only your life, but those closest to you?

_____

_____

_____

_____

_____

_____

3. How did it feel going to bed at your designated time? (To be answered after you take the challenge.)

_____

_____

_____

_____

_____

_____

_____

Day 19

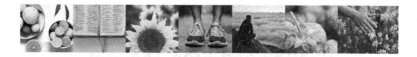

Prioritizing Rest

*By the seventh day God had finished the work he
had been doing; so on the seventh day he rested
from all his work. Then God blessed the seventh
day and made it holy, because on it he rested from
all the work of creating that he had done.*
—Genesis 2:2-3 NIV

Most of us are familiar with the story of creation. God created the
world and everything in it in a matter of six days. This doesn't come
as a shock to many of us, because He is God, after all. He can do anything He wants to at any moment. What does come as a shock is that
on the seventh day, He rested. God, the creator of the universe, rested.
Many have asked the question of why God chose to rest. I don't believe
the reason is because He grew tired and *had* to rest, but rather He
wanted to show us the importance and beauty behind resting.

Rest doesn't have to look like a good night's sleep or a midday nap;
however, those are both great ways to rest! Rest often includes doing
things that you enjoy. Rest could look like going for a long walk or
hike, having brunch with a friend, reading a good book, or taking a
long bath. Rest is anything that helps bring peace to your mind and
body. Rest helps send the message to your body, soul, and spirit that
you're honoring and loving yourself in the best ways possible.

As you go throughout your day today, ask yourself what rest looks like to you. Try to incorporate one or more things into your day that will help rejuvenate your mind, body, and soul.

Healthy and Free Thought

Rest is so important to God that even He chose to rest! Rest is what brings harmony to our body, soul, and spirit. Resting has the ability to help heal and calm our bodies.

Time to Reflect

1. What are some realistic ways you can incorporate taking time to rest into your life?

_____

_____

_____

_____

_____

2. Why do you think that rest is so important to God?

_____

_____

_____

_____

_____

_____

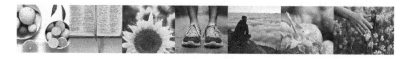

Sleeping through the Storm

But soon a fierce storm came up. High waves were breaking into the boat, and it began to fill with water. Jesus was sleeping at the back of the boat with his head on a cushion. The disciples woke him up, shouting, "Teacher, don't you care that we're going to drown?" When Jesus woke up, he rebuked the wind and said to the waves, "Silence! Be still!" Suddenly the wind stopped, and there was a great calm.

—MARK 4:37-39

Perhaps one of the most perfect examples of someone who lived from a place of rest is Jesus. He had the highest calling on His life in the history of the world and very easily could have fallen prey to the pressures of stress and performance. But He knew who He was and who His Father called Him to be and, therefore, made the decision to live from a place of rest.

A perfect example of this is found in Mark chapter 4. After a day of preaching to crowds, Jesus and His disciples decide to go to the other side of the lake. On their journey, a storm broke loose and sent His disciples into a state of fear and chaos as the boat began to fill with water. When they found Jesus, He was *asleep* in the midst of the storm. After being awakened by His disciples, He simply spoke to the winds and commanded them to stop. Sure enough, the storm passed and the waters were calm once again. This is a beautiful picture of how Jesus carried and lived from such a place of rest that even His words carried authority over any storm. He simply released what was already within Him.

As Christians, we are called to live from a place of rest. Rest is where breakthrough is formed and brought forth. When we live from a place of rest, we then carry peace and use it to change the atmosphere around us—much like Jesus did.

Today's challenge is to find that place of rest within yourself. When you feel that your circumstances or environment are beginning to cause chaos around you, ask yourself what Jesus thinks of the situation and then declare His word over the environment. Believe that because you live from a place of peace, you can change the world around you.

Healthy and Free Thought

We were created and designed to live from a place of rest. Doing so allows us to bring peace not only to ourselves, but to those around us.

Time to Reflect

1. What does living from a place of rest look like from a kingdom perspective?

_____

_____

_____

_____

_____

_____

_____

2. Jesus spent His life studying, traveling, and teaching and yet He still was able to live from a place of rest. What steps can you take to make sure your peace is changing the atmosphere around you...and not the other way around?

_____

_____

_____

_____

_____

_____

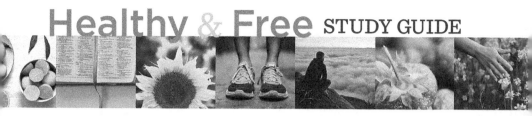

Session 5

Movement

Many years ago, my chiropractor said to me, "Our bodies were made to move." How many of us can attest to that? Probably everyone has experienced those days when you sit on the couch for hours watching television only to feel stagnant, over-tired, and a little foggy-brained. Once we stand up and begin to move around, we start to feel better. We really were not meant to be sedentary creatures. The goal is to find something that you enjoy so that exercise doesn't become a chore. Whether it's lifting weights for an hour at the gym, going for a bike ride, or pressing play to work out with a YouTube Pilates video, just do it!

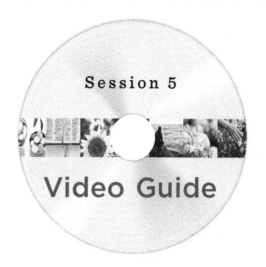

Session 5

Video Guide

1. You were created to _____.

2. Muscle trains your brain to _____ your bones.

3. Find out what kind of movement fits your _____ and start moving!

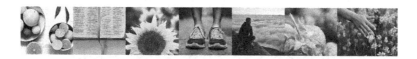

Weekly Health Practice

Get moving! Your body was created to move, so find ways that you can start moving every day!

Note about Session 5

Today's session is going to be unique, as I will be demonstrating some easy-to-do exercises. Whether you belong to a gym, are interested in buying some at-home gym equipment, or simply want to find some form of movement that best suits your present lifestyle, this session is designed to give you a quick glimpse of a few exercises that might be helpful to you. The goal is *not* to make you feel like you need to go out and sign up for a monthly gym membership or make an expensive purchase of exercise equipment. Instead, ask your journey companion, the Holy Spirit, what form of movement would be suit *this unique place* on your journey.

Discussion Questions

The questions will be limited today, as the focus will be more on the activation component.

- Why is building muscle so important? What will this do?

- What are some things you can start doing in your everyday life to start moving?

- Have group members share their stories of how they started moving (just like the woman I mentioned who started swimming).

Activation Exercise: Start Moving!

Get together in small groups and discuss some practical ways that you can start moving. The goal is for each participant to come up with *one* thing that he or she can incorporate into the everyday routine to increase movement.

Use the space below to brainstorm some ways you can start moving:

_____

_____

_____

_____

_____

_____

_____

_____

_____

_____

_____

_____

_____

_____

_____

_____

_____

_____

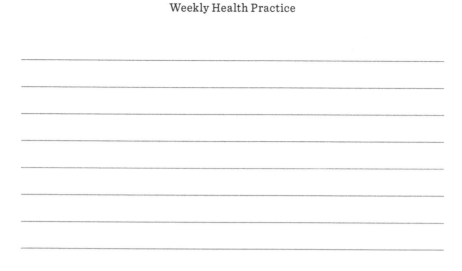

After 10-15 minutes, come back together and present your different ideas before the whole group/class.

Once again, the goal is to identify *one* method of movement that you can begin incorporating into everyday life—regardless of how busy or demanding your schedule is or how much time you spend at an office desk, inside.

The key is beginning with something that easily works with your present schedule. Soon enough, as you see the benefits that movement has on your overall health, you will begin to *schedule around* movement (this might be joining a gym, running, bicycling, playing a sport, etc.).

Don't feel like you need to start at a gym to get moving. The goal is not to start big, but to start *somewhere*!

Today, figure out what you are going to do *this week* to start moving!

Weekly Exercises

Engage your weekly activities in the study guide. While doing so, try to practice your movement every day. Even if it's just for a short time, the consistency is very important.

You can find more information about movement in Chapter 4 of the *Healthy and Free* book.

Day 21

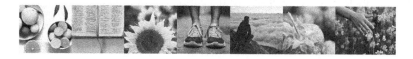

One Small Step

He gives strength to the weary and
increases the power of the weak.
—Isaiah 40:29 NIV

When making the change toward a healthy lifestyle, you cannot escape the exercise component. In today's culture, many of us lead very sedentary lives. We drive to work, spend most of our day sitting down, and go home exhausted only to sit down in front of the television all night. So, when it comes to exercise, the thought can be overwhelming. Thoughts of marathon running and boot camp style workouts come plaguing the mind, and many give up before they even start. However, today is the day that changes.

As with any journey, it all begins with one step. I want you to forget what prejudices you may have about exercise, any excuses, or any fears and just start. Many of us can come up with a long list of valid reasons why we *can't* exercise; however, we can always make time for what is important to us. It may look like taking a ten-minute walk, doing some jumping jacks, or starting to train for that 5K you've been wanting to do for years. Whatever it is, today is your day to begin that journey.

Our bodies were designed to move. So exercise is just another way that we can love, honor, and steward the body that God gave us. When beginning a new exercise routine, remembering your *why* is going to help get you through those moments when you feel like skipping out on a workout. However, keeping that vision will help keep you motivated.

Healthy and Free Thought

Our bodies were made for exercise! Pushing past our excuses and moving forward will not only honor our bodies, but will strengthen our minds.

Time to Reflect

1. What is a practical way I can incorporate fitness into my daily life?

_____

_____

_____

_____

_____

_____

2. What are the long-term benefits of adding exercise to my life?

_____

_____

_____

_____

_____

_____

3. How will remembering my why help me get motivated to get moving?

_____

_____

_____

_____

_____

_____

Day 22

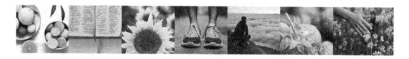

Adjusting Your Mindset

*Whether you think you can or you
think you can't—you're right.*
—Henry Ford

Most of us, at one time or another have said: "I hate exercise!" It's uncomfortable, challenging, and at times painful. Why would anyone want to willingly make themselves go through that kind of pain? And better yet, what is wrong with those people who actually *love* to exercise?

The difference between the people who love to exercise and the people who detest it is that the people who love it decided to adjust their mindset. You see, when we partner with a thought like, "I hate exercise," we actually give that thought power and it becomes our truth.

So next time you find yourself lacing up your shoes with dread, I want you to intentionally adjust your mindset. Instead of thinking that you *have* to exercise, switch your thinking to you *get* to exercise. There are many people out there who have physical disabilities or have lost an arm, leg, or both who would do anything to be able to have and steward the body that *you* have.

Today, I challenge you to adjust your thinking when it comes to exercise. Whether you are taking a walk, lifting weights, swimming, or having quality time on the elliptical, continuously pray this prayer: "*God, thank You for the body that You have given me. Thank You that I have the health and ability to take care of my body and use it for Your glory."*

Healthy and Free Thought

Learning to enjoy exercise and movement all begins in the mind. Intentionally adjusting my mindset will lead to greater breakthrough.

Time to Reflect

1.   How will adjusting my mindset help me push toward my health goals?

_____

_____

_____

_____

_____

_____

2.   What are some positive declarations I can begin to speak over myself that are related to exercise? (List three.)

_____

_____

_____

_____

_____

_____

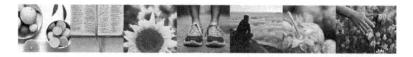

Discover Your Potential

I can do all things through Christ who strengthens me.
—PHILIPPIANS 4:13 NKJV

Whenever we start something that may be foreign to us, like exercise, it is easy to compare our beginning to other people's end. Many times, we are so quick to discredit the ability that we have. Sometimes, it takes having another person believing in us to help push us beyond our comfort level and into a new level of greatness. This same principle is true for exercise. A common thought among those who begin working out is, "I never thought that I could do this!"

A great way to discover your potential is to enlist a friend or family member to be your cheerleader! People often even see a greater success rate when they find a workout partner or personal trainer to help keep them accountable during those times when going to the gym feels so unappealing. Having that accountability will help unleash your potential.

Next time you are tempted to rob yourself of your potential by skipping a weight lifting rep or jumping off the treadmill five minutes early, remember *why* you are on this journey to begin with. Ask the Holy Spirit to help guide you and give you strength to endure during your workouts. Remember, you can do all things through Him.

Healthy and Free Challenge

Ask the Holy Spirit to show you who you can ask in your life to come alongside you in this journey. Once He reveals that to you, reach out and ask them to be your cheerleader or even join you through this journey.

Time to Reflect

1. How will inviting another trusted friend or family member help me on this journey to health and wellness?

_____

_____

_____

_____

_____

_____

2. When I feel like giving up, what quote or Bible verse can I use to help remind me of why I started in the first place?

_____

_____

_____

_____

_____

_____

Day 24

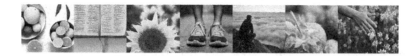

Find Your Vision

I've got my eye on the goal, where God is beckoning us onward—to Jesus. I'm off and running, and I'm not turning back. So let's keep focused on that goal, those of us who want everything God has for us.
—Philippians 3:14-15 MSG

Yesterday we discussed the importance of discovering your potential and finding someone to help cheer you on during this journey. Another key part in discovering your potential is going to come from having a vision, or a goal for yourself when it comes to fitness. Without a goal, you will find it almost impossible to wake up early for a workout or log miles on a treadmill. Skipping out on a workout becomes far too easy when we don't take into consideration the negative impact it would have on our goals.

As Christians, many of us are used to having spiritual disciplines because we have a long-term goal ahead that we work toward. We read our Bible to strengthen ourselves in His word, we pray to grow closer to God, and we go to church because we want to grow in community and feed our spirits. It is now time for the church to use that same principle and apply it toward our health and fitness.

The key to seeing yourself reach your goals is to have one long-term goal and a variety of short-term goals leading up to it. Let's say your goal is to run a marathon and that's the only goal you have set. If you aren't used to running, then that goal is going to overwhelm you when you first try to go on a run and can't make it to a mile. Instead, set a goal to run half a mile, then one mile, then two miles, then five. Each time you reach your short-term goal, you'll beam with pride and eventually you'll find yourself reaching your long-term goal.

Healthy and Free Challenge

Having a goal for ourselves will help give us a vision to work toward. When we can see how each step plays into the biggest picture, it makes it far harder to try to give up!

Time to Reflect

1. How will having a goal help motivate me to stay on this fitness journey?

_____

_____

_____

_____

_____

_____

_____

2. What long-term goal do I have that I want to see myself reach? (Don't be afraid to dream big!)

_____

_____

_____

_____

_____

_____

_____

_____

_____

3. What are some short-term goals that I can implement that will
    help me eventually reach my long-term goal?

_____

_____

_____

_____

_____

_____

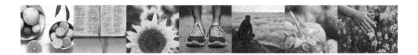

Giving Yourself Grace

*I'm not saying that I have this all together, that I have
it made. But I am well on my way, reaching out for
Christ, who has so wondrously reached out for me.*
—PHILIPPIANS 3:12 MSG

Remember, push yourself to discover your fullest potential, but celebrate your successes along the way!

Healthy and Free Thought

Grace is an important concept especially in the process of adjusting to a healthy lifestyle. Remember, this is a journey meaning that there may be some mess-ups and wrong turns along the way. Grace is going to allow us to get back on track without missing a beat.

Time to Reflect

1. Has there been a time when I didn't allow myself grace in a certain situation? How did that affect my overall being and motivation?

_____

_____

_____

_____

_____

_____

_____

_____

2.   How will incorporating grace into my lifestyle help keep me on
     my journey to health and wellness?

_____

_____

_____

_____

_____

_____

_____

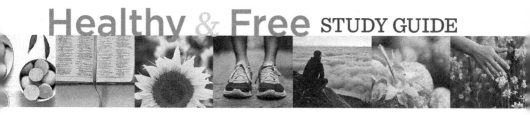

Session 6

Having Fun with Food

People are often surprised when they hear how passionate I am about food and especially when I tell them that I eat a lot. In fact, over the years this is one of the secrets that I have learned in maintaining a healthy weight for my size and age. Through my own experience and watching countless friends struggle, I have come to believe that one of the systemic problems in the diet industry is the persistent over-emphasis on low-calorie eating or what I call "glorified starvation diets." I want to encourage you to recognize these triggers, stop dieting, and start nourishing your body with healthy, organic, living foods.

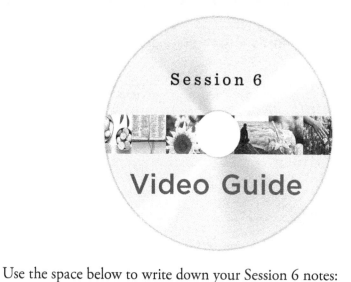

Session 6

Video Guide

Use the space below to write down your Session 6 notes:

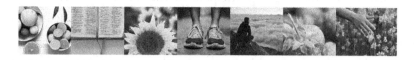

Weekly Health Practice

Eat clean! Because food is meant to be enjoyed, the key to eating well is putting the right kinds of foods into your body.

Discussion Questions

1. What did you find most surprising about what I shared about eating and diet?

2. Prepare to share your personal experiences with dieting versus completely changing the way you eat. How can dieting be negative?

3. List some practical ways you can start eating healthy right now.

4. Once you begin changing the way you eat, what are some ways you can "maneuver" through a restaurant menu?

5. Share your journey to eating well. What simple steps did you take to start changing your eating habits? (The goal is to make it simple and executable.)

Activation Exercise

Changing the way you eat doesn't have to be difficult!

Take this time to brainstorm in small groups and come up with a one-step process to *start* eating right. The goal is taking baby steps, not necessarily trying to quit something "cold turkey."

The problem with most diets is that they are overcomplicated. The goal here is not to simply participate in the latest fad diet for a season—only going back to eating like "normal" afterward. The goal is to change your way of eating and come up with a new normal.

Based on what I shared in Session 6, what is *one thing* you can start doing that will help you eat better?

This can be anything from:

- Finding healthy replacements for sugar and sweets

- Buying certain foods organic

- Progressively getting rid of some foods that are harmful to your diet

During this time, I encourage you to:

- Be creative.

- Make a list.

- Learn from each other.

- Be sure to ask plenty of questions—especially to other participants who have already made some of these changes and are experiencing success.

Weekly Exercises

Engage your weekly activities in the study guide. While doing so, try to practice your movement every day. Even if it's just for a short time, the consistency is very important.

You can find more information about healthy eating habits and tips in Chapter 4 of the *Healthy and Free* book.

Day 26

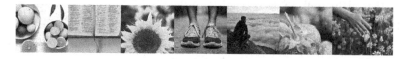

An Honest Assessment

So, whether you eat or drink, or whatever
you do, do all to the glory of God.
—1 Corinthians 10:31 ESV

Ahhh, food. The smell, the taste, and the memories associated with it all strike a chord with each one of us in one way or another. We live in a culture where food is used in almost every occasion and life season. If something positive happens to you, like a promotion or an engagement, you celebrate with friends over food. If you lose a family member or friend, you mourn with friends over food. Food is perhaps the only thing that every person has in common because we all have to eat to live. Because of that, it is nearly impossible to walk 50 feet in any major city without passing at least three restaurants, a food stand, and a coffee shop.

Because of our abundance of food and our busy schedules, many of us have become oblivious to the amount and quality of food we are eating. It's easy to fly through our days scarfing down a large coffee and a breakfast burrito for breakfast, followed by a stale scone for lunch, and end the day mindlessly eating an entire bag of chips and yet still feel like we didn't eat anything the entire day! Food is far too good to be wasted by mindless eating!

Today's challenge is to take an honest inventory of your day-to-day eating habits. A good way to do this is to keep a log of everything you eat and drink from the moment you wake up to the moment you go to bed. You may be surprised by what you see! This challenge isn't meant to make you feel guilty or to cast shame on anyone, but it will help shed a light on where you may need to be willing to make some changes in order to meet your goals. Sometimes it takes becoming completely honest with ourselves before we can see the need for change in our own lives.

Healthy and Free Thought

It is easy to go through our days either eating too much food or not enough. Taking an honest assessment, even if painful, will be the first step in seeing what changes need to be made.

Time to Reflect

1. What practical change can I begin to incorporate today that will help me reach my goals?

_____

_____

_____

_____

_____

_____

2. Why is it important to take an honest assessment of our day-to-day food choices and how can this help impact my journey for the better?

_____

_____

_____

_____

_____

_____

_____

_____

_____

_____

_____

_____

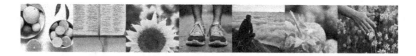

Changing Your Mind

*I appeal to you therefore, brothers, by the mercies of
God, to present your bodies as a living sacrifice, holy
and acceptable to God, which is your spiritual worship.*
—ROMANS 12:1 ESV

We've previously discussed in both Session 2: "Soul Health" and Session 5: "Movement" how making the decision to change your mind is crucial to seeing success in those areas. The same is true when it comes to changing the way we eat. As with any change, it will often take reminding ourselves of our *why* when we feel like giving up. Food is now used to comfort and pleasure rather than to fuel our bodies in today's culture. So changing your mindset in regard to food may take diligence on your part.

When making the decision to embark on a new lifestyle, changing your mind about food and your food choices may be the most difficult change. If you were raised without being taught the importance of nutrition, it will oftentimes feel like you are re-learning how to live in this area. There will be times when you'll be tempted to reach for a pint of ice cream after a log day, but with time and practice you will have the power to overcome those temptations!

A key to changing your mind is remembering that you are powerful! Food does not control you! You have the ability to make good choices that honor both your body and your future in every situation you face. It can be challenging when you're out with your friends while they scarf down nachos and pizza. In those moments, it's easy to make excuses and tell yourself that you'll just start again tomorrow, and in some cases that is okay. The goal is not to live a life of deprivation. But before you decide to join them instead of opting for a fresh salad, remind yourself of your why. That will give a purpose behind your choosing to say no in that moment. Remember that when you say no in that moment, you are actually saying yes to your why.

Remembering your why is going to be what gets you through the tough days and nights. Instead of embracing the depravation mentality, remind yourself that the food you are eating is actually bringing life to every cell in your body! You are healing yourself from the inside out! Some moments may take more mindful discipline than others, but over time you will find that it gets easier and easier and your taste buds and your body would much prefer the healthier food options.

Healthy and Free Thought

You are powerful over food! The key to seeing lasting change in your diet is to remember your why and make the intentional decision to change your mind about the way you see food.

Time to Reflect

1. When it comes to eating healthy, do I feel deprived or revived? How can I switch those feelings of deprivation to ones of celebration?

_____

_____

2. How will adjusting the way I think about food help further me
    on my journey?

_____

_____

_____

_____

_____

_____

3. What positive affirmations can I speak over myself when I am
    tempted to throw in the towel on healthy eating?

_____

_____

_____

_____

_____

_____

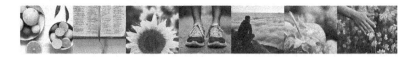

Making the Switch

And let us not grow weary of doing good, for in
due season we will reap, if we do not give up.
—GALATIANS 6:9 ESV

In a world where it seems that a new diet presents itself every week, it can be difficult to navigate and find what works the best for you. If there was just one magic diet, everyone would be on it and this series would not be needed! But the truth is, there isn't a real quick fix or a "one size fits all" when it comes to eating.

For one, dieting is not the answer. Dieting is a short-term fix that many times leads to failure because it is unrealistic. To see lasting change, we need to let go of the diet mentality and embrace a new way of eating. When changing our eating habits, it is tempting to want to go into it 100 percent, which for some works well. For most, making lasting change is more of a step-by-step process.

Take a moment to imagine what your ideal diet would look like. I imagine that it would be filled with life-giving fruits and vegetables, quality proteins, and hearty whole grains. The key to getting there is by taking one day at a time. If you have been a fast-food addict, having the expectation to become a health guru in a week is not realistic! It will take some exploring and experimenting with food. Practice paying attention to your body as you incorporate more healthy foods into your diet and see if you notice any changes in the way it feels and functions.

You'll find that some foods will give you more energy and others may not. Some people function well on a low or zero grain diet, while others need grains to feel good. There is no way of knowing what works best for you until you try!

While making the switch to a healthy lifestyle, the mistake most people make is cutting out their "guilty pleasures" all at once. Quitting sugar, soda, and processed foods cold turkey is a recipe for disaster especially when it is all you have ever known. A more realistic approach is to choose to eliminate one thing at a time. Remember, we are not on this journey to find a quick fix. Doing this may take more time in the long run, but you will find yourself to be so much more successful.

As you go through your day, ask yourself what steps you can begin to implement in your diet that will help you reach your goals.

Healthy and Free Thought

In order to make a lasting change, we must be willing to give up the diet mentality and embrace the process of change. Perfection is not the expectation.

Time to Reflect

1. What small changes can I begin implementing that will be realistic for helping me on this journey?

---

2. How will making small, lasting changes be different from the "all or nothing" mentality I may be used to?

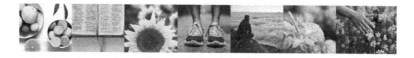

Healing from the Inside Out

And God said, "Behold, I have given you every plant
yielding seed that is on the face of all the earth, and every
tree with seed in its fruit. You shall have them for food."
—Genesis 1:29 ESV

God is nothing short of a genius, especially when it comes to His idea of food. He could have created something bland for us to use for energy, but instead He created a vast array of food ranging from fresh fruits to colorful vegetables to satisfying grains. He created food to be pleasurable, enjoyable, and fun!

Not only did He create a variety for taste, but He also created food to help keep us healthy and help us heal from the inside out. For example, many of us love the use of garlic, especially in Italian dishes or when paired with butter. But did you know that garlic acts as a natural antibiotic when ingested as well as reduces inflammation and has cardio protective benefits?[1] It is a powerful and natural medicine that many of us already have in our homes!

Creating a diet that is rich in fruits and vegetables is not just about keeping calories at a minimum. It is about aiding our body in its day-to-day work as well as bringing natural healing to our bodies. One of the many reasons that people begin to feel great after adding more plant-based foods into their diets is because they are flooding their body with vitamins and minerals that it needs to survive!

So next time you find yourself tempted to order take-out rather than make a healthy homemade meal at home, remind yourself of all the ways your body will thank you if you choose the latter. Today your challenge is to do a bit of research on the health benefits of the foods that you are putting into your body. It will make eating healthy so much more exciting and satisfying!

Healthy and Free Thought

God intended us to eat a diet rich in plant-based foods as a way to help supplement and love our bodies from the inside out!

Time to Reflect

1. When I consider all the vitamins and minerals that are found in plant-based foods, how does that motivate me to want to make healthier choices?

_____

_____

_____

_____

_____

_____

_____

_____

2. After researching the benefits of the foods I am using to nourish my body, how does that change my perception of healthy foods?

_____

_____

_____

_____

_____

_____

_____

_____

Note

1. The George Mateljan Foundation, "Garlic," The World's Healthiest Foods, accessed April 18, 2015, http://www.whfoods.com/genpage.php?tname=foodspice&dbid=60.

Day 30

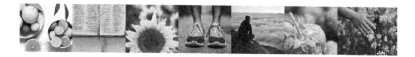

Grace

Jesus replied: "'Love the Lord your God with all your heart and with all your soul and with all your mind.' This is the first and greatest commandment. And the second is like it: 'Love your neighbor as yourself.' All the Law and the Prophets hang on these two commandments."
—Matthew 22:37-40 NIV

As you may have already encountered, this journey is going to be filled with some wandering and wrong turns. The beauty of this journey is that the goal is not perfection. A bad day doesn't mean failure. It just means that you have the decision to either stand back up or stay down.

When it comes to re-learning how to eat properly and adjusting our lifestyle, it's easy to make mistakes, overeat at times, or make a choice that doesn't help us. The key is to learn from those moments and embrace them as a chance to reflect and grow from it. There are also going to be moments that are beyond our control. I recall a time when I was traveling through the South and was given a plate of foods that I would normally not consider eating. However, I chose to eat them, living from a place of grace, not perfection.

The topic of grace is covered a few times through this study because its importance cannot be stressed enough. Grace is going to be what covers, protects, and leads us back to a place of wholeness.

So, if you've fallen over a few times, give yourself grace. You are not alone. This is a journey that you were created for.

Healthy and Free Thought

Grace is a repeated topic throughout this study because it is vital to our success. The journey to health and wellness is ongoing and at times unpredictable. Operating from a place of grace allows us to continue to grow despite obstacles.

Time to Reflect

1. How do I normally respond when I "mess up" whether it's in my diet or in life?

_____

_____

_____

_____

_____

_____

2. How will learning to operate from a place of grace help change the outcome of my journey?

_____

_____

_____

_____

_____

_____

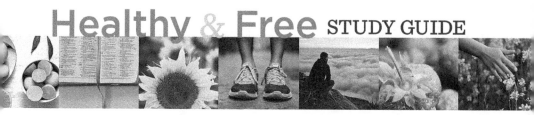
Session 7

The Skinny Obsession

"Hunger took my pain away. The ache in my stomach distracted me from the pain in my heart. I could control my hunger pangs, which in a funny way made me feel powerful when I couldn't control the emotional pain that I was feeling."

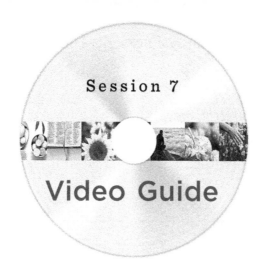

Session 7

Video Guide

Use the space below to write down your Session 7 notes:

_____

_____

_____

_____

_____

_____

_____

_____

_____

_____

_____

_____

_____

_____

_____

_____

_____

_____

_____

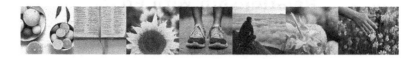

Weekly Health Practice

Instead of turning to food for emotional support, try at least two new coping skills to get you through a difficult day or moment. Get creative and have fun!

Discussion Questions (25-30 Minutes)

1. What are some signs that we can be aware of that will show us if we have allowed food to have an unhealthy place in our lives?

2. Describe what food addiction could look like. Have you ever recognized food taking an unhealthy place in your life? How were you able to overcome that?

3. How will learning to cultivate a healthy body image help break any chains that food addiction has used to keep us in bondage?

4. What are some healthy non-food related coping skills we can incorporate into our lives to help manage stress?

5. How does food addiction create a disconnect from ourselves and the people around us in our lives?

6. Discuss how healthy coping skills bring strength to our lives.

Activation: Evaluate Your Relationship with Food

This is an exercise for you to engage in *individually*.

1. Ask the Holy Spirit to reveal to you any ways you have allowed food to comfort you. How has turning to food created a disconnect in your heart?

2. Ask the Holy Spirit to reveal new coping skills that you can use in difficult situations. It can be calling a friend, going for a walk, or taking a long bath. Find at least ten healthy coping skills that you will be able to choose from when you find yourself wanting to turn to food for comfort.

You can write these out in the space below:

_____

_____

_____

_____

_____

_____

_____

_____

_____

_____

_____

_____

_____

_____

_____

_____

_____

_____

_____

_____

_____

_____

_____

_____

_____

_____

_____

_____

_____

_____

_____

_____

_____

Weekly Exercises

Work to become aware of how you respond to stress. Do you suddenly crave chocolate or fried foods if you've had a hard day? Or is it after a sleepless night? When you find yourself wanting to reach for your chocolate stash, choose something from your list of coping skills before turning to food.

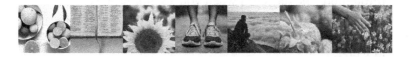

Identifying Food Addiction

Now the Lord is the Spirit, and where the
Spirit of the Lord is, there is freedom.
—2 CORINTHIANS 3:17 NIV

A topic that many people do not feel comfortable discussing is food addiction. It is estimated that 24 million Americans associate themselves with having an eating disorder and 8 million claim to struggle with binge eating in particular.[1] This is a serious and even at times a fatal issue that is kept secret because it often brings feelings of shame and low self-esteem.

Food addiction goes beyond the occasional night when you over-indulge in your favorite meal or dessert. It is often an obsession that leads to one feeling out of control when it comes to food. Feelings of hopelessness and constant defeat can oftentimes feel overwhelming for those struggling.

Second Corinthians 3:17 says that *"where the Spirit of the Lord is, there is freedom."* Jesus didn't give His life for you to be a slave to food! If you struggle with food addiction, be encouraged knowing that God wants to see you free more than you want to be free!

Food addiction can manifest itself in the form of anorexia, bulimia, and binge eating disorders. A good way to decipher if you have a food addiction is to ask yourself these questions:

1. Do you find yourself obsessing over what you are going to eat throughout the day even when you are not hungry?

2. Do you try to eat healthy in public but eat large amounts of food in secret?

3. When you begin to eat an "unhealthy" food, do you feel out of control and unable to stop?

If you answered yes to one or more of these questions, you may have a food addiction. Don't be afraid to seek help from a friend or a medical professional. If you struggle with food addiction, I invite you to pray this prayer:

> *Father, I repent for believing the lie that I am unable to overcome this food addiction. I believe that Your Son died so that I may be free and I declare that this is my day of freedom. I let go of food addiction and I say that you no longer serve a purpose in me. I receive the gift of grace and unconditional love that the Father offers me. I believe that through Christ, I am powerful and free from addiction.*

Healthy and Free Thought

We were not created to live as slaves to food. Living with a food addiction should not bring shame, but hope knowing that there is freedom.

Time to Reflect

1. What would it look like to be free from a food addiction?

_____

_____

_____

_____

_____

_____

_____

2. If you struggle with a food addiction, take the time to ask the Lord what steps you should take to overcome it. Journal your answer here.

_____

_____

_____

_____

_____

_____

3. If you want to feel stretched, challenge yourself to share your struggle with a trusted family member or friend and ask them to speak truth into your life regarding your situation. After doing so, write down what truths they were able to speak into your life regarding it.

_____

_____

_____

_____

_____

_____

Note

1. "Binge Eating Disorder," ANAD, accessed April 18, 2015, http://www
   .anad.org/get-information/about-eating-disorders/binge-eating
   -disorder/.

Day 32

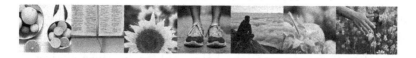

Finding Comfort in Food

All praise to God, the Father of our Lord Jesus Christ.
God is our merciful Father and the source of all comfort.
—2 CORINTHIANS 1:3

In this day and age, it is not uncommon for many people to go to food for comfort. Many of us were raised with food being a reward system. When we were hurt, our parents gave us a lollipop. When you had your tonsils out, people brought you ice cream. When you had a bad day, your mom may have made you your favorite meal to help bring you joy. When this happens, the message that food is a reward and will make you feel better is constantly being reinforced, and many then grow up wondering why they automatically crave chocolate or fatty foods the moment something goes wrong in their life.

To an extent, the idea of food bringing comfort is not wrong. Food is meant to be enjoyed and savored. It only becomes a problem when it becomes our only source of comfort in this life.

The problem with food being our source of comfort is that it is unfulfilling. It brings temporary relief from the pain because it only serves as a distraction. Once our plate is empty or the pint of ice cream is gone, the fear and anxiety that we were trying to suppress comes bubbling back up to the surface. Oftentimes, this can lead to binging if one does not want to face what they are feeling on the inside.

It is possible to be an emotional eater without even realizing it. Oftentimes, some people feel that there are no emotions attached to their constant overeating because they have stuffed their feelings down so deep within them they are almost numb to them. It often becomes evident that there are emotions being hidden by their choices when they are forced to change their lifestyle. Being afraid to feel their emotions will often knock them off the straight and narrow and back into their old habits. Don't be afraid of your emotions. They are often trying to communicate with us that something is wrong within us and we need to be able to see it to speak truth to it.

As with any habit, you have the ability to change how you respond to what you may be feeling. If you catch yourself reaching for a bag of chips after having a fight with a friend or family member, stop and remind yourself of your why. If you are unsure why you are wanting to binge or overeat, it can be helpful to take an inventory of what just happened that lead up to that point. Ask yourself, *did anything happen today that has caused me to feel unsafe? Did I get my feelings hurt? Did I say or do something hurtful to someone else? How does my body feel? Am I overtired or over worked? Is this something just some rest could fix?*

Sometimes events happen so quickly that we may not have even realized how a certain comment may have affected us or how hurtful that fight with a loved one may have been. Once you are able to narrow down what is driving you to want to turn to food for comfort, remind yourself of your why. *Why* are you going to opt out of stuffing your emotions? You can then still do something to help nurture yourself. It may look different than you are used to like a warm bath, a long walk, or some quiet time with God. It will feel uncomfortable at first because it will be different than what you are used to, but over time you will begin to feel so much more freedom and peace over your circumstances.

For some of you reading this, you may already know that you are an emotional eater. But for others it may be unclear. Take a moment to pause and ask the Holy Spirit what He sees that you may not be seeing and be open to what He has to say. Remember, He is on your side.

Healthy and Free Thought

God wants to be our comforter, so when we turn to food instead of turning to Him we are robbing Him of that opportunity. Learning to steward and feel our emotions in a healthy way is going to bring us to a place of freedom and peace.

Time to Reflect

1. Take a moment to ask the Holy Spirit where your heart is emotionally. If you struggle with emotional eating, ask Him to reveal to you what emotions or memories you may be trying to avoid. If you are unsure if you struggle with emotional eating, simply ask the Holy Spirit to reveal that to you.

_____

_____

_____

_____

_____

_____

2. If you struggle with emotional eating, what emotions or painful memories did the Holy Spirit reveal to you that you may be trying to avoid?

_____

_____

_____

_____

_____

_____

_____

3. How will being brave and willing to face my emotions positively impact my life and future?

_____

_____

_____

_____

_____

_____

4. What three things can I do to help nurture myself in times of distress instead of turning to food?

_____

_____

_____

_____

_____

_____

Day 33

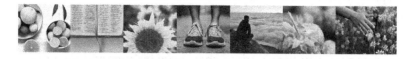

Speaking to Your Emotions

Be strong, courageous, and firm; fear not nor be in
terror before them, for it is the Lord your God Who
goes with you; He will not fail you or forsake you.
—DEUTERONOMY 31:6 AMP

Yesterday we discussed emotional eating and ways to help overcome it. Today we are going to dig a little deeper and learn how to communicate with our emotions.

Part of the disconnect that happens between the body, soul, and spirit takes place during times of discomfort, trauma, or stress. Pain and negative feelings hurt and we have been wired to avoid it. In the natural, it makes sense. If you are sick, you go to the doctor so he or she can give you medicine to take the pain away. If you scrape your knee as a child, you run to your mother for a bandage and a kiss to make it feel better. Pain just doesn't feel good, plain and simple.

The same is true when it comes to emotional pain. The problem with emotional pain is that there isn't an over-the-counter drug or bandage that can fix it for us. If we are unwilling to deal with it, the only other option is to distract ourselves from it. Many choose food, others choose drugs, some choose alcohol, and the list goes on and on. When we do this, it's like trying to use duct tape to shut down a tornado. It just doesn't work without getting sucked into the tornado ourselves.

Emotions are not bad. They are simply a way that our body, soul, and spirit choose to communicate to one another. Learning to be okay with your feelings is going to be a key to helping you live a healthy and free life. If you've been an emotional eater or have some buried hurts from your past, you have noticed that those feelings and memories have begun to come to the surface as you've done this study. This is completely normal, as the Lord wants to see you deal with them so that they no longer have bondage over you. Instead of trying to push them down once again, I am going to encourage you to speak to your emotions.

If you did yesterday's reflection questions, you asked the Holy Spirit to reveal to you what emotions or memories you may be trying to avoid. I want you to remember those emotions He revealed to you and use the outline below to address them:

> (Your Name) *I am sorry for not allowing you to feel the things that were going on in your heart. I repent for not listening to you when you were trying to communicate with me. I give you permission to feel and to experience the depth of your heart. There is no need to be afraid of feelings and emotions because God is your comfort and your protector. He will never let you go.*
>
> *I speak to (emotion) and I no longer need you to protect me because God is my protector. Psalm 23 says, "The Lord is my shepherd; I have all that I need. He lets me rest in green meadows; he leads me beside peaceful streams. He renews my strength. He guides me along right paths, bringing honor to his name." I hold close to the promises of God trusting that He holds me close.*

You can use this outline throughout your journey when painful emotions begin arising within you. This can also be used to address lies you've believed about yourself, addictive patterns you may have, or fears that keep bubbling to the surface. Remember that speaking the living word of God over ourselves brings more hope and healing in a moment than self-protection can in a lifetime.

Healthy and Free Thought

Negative emotions are not bad or created to hurt you. They are normally there to communicate with you that something is off in your heart and needs attention. Being willing to allow ourselves to feel those emotions and replacing them with truth is vital to becoming healthy and free.

Time to Reflect

1. Are emotions and feelings something that I used to run from in the past?

_____

_____

_____

_____

_____

_____

_____

2. How will acknowledging what my heart is feeling help me on this journey to health and wellness?

_____

_____

_____

_____

_____

_____

_____

Day 34

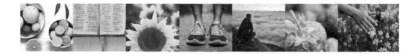

Creating a Healthy Relationship with Food

One should eat to live, not live to eat.
—BENJAMIN FRANKLIN

Now that we've walked through what having a food addiction looks like and addressed the issues that may be associated with it, we can begin to create a healthy relationship with food.

Many people who have attempted to lose weight countless times in the past create an unhealthy relationship with food. When food begins serving a purpose other than being used for fuel, it can turn into something unhealthy. For example, for someone who struggles with anorexia or bulimia, food is often feared and seen as something that can potentially hurt and destroy them. For someone who struggles with binge eating, food can be feared but also used to suppress fear. For a chronic dieter, food often feels overpowering and makes the dieter feel powerless. All of these traits carry an unhealthy relationship with food because the food is being given power that it was never meant to have.

Let's take a look at what food is. *Webster's Dictionary* defines it as "material consisting essentially of protein, carbohydrate, and fat used in the body of an organism to sustain growth, repair, and vital processes and to furnish energy." Notice that it does not say that it has the power to make someone love you more or less, give you your dream job, or guarantee you tomorrow. As funny as that may sound, many of us have given it that same amount of power.

How many of us have opted out of a night out with friends because we ate too much the week prior? A simple decision like that shows that you may have an unhealthy relationship with food. You've given food the power to decide whether or not you are going to feel good about yourself. You've given food the ability to dictate how the people in your life are going to experience you.

A way to create a healthy relationship with food is to intentionally eliminate any good or bad feelings associated with it. For example, if you put all your self-esteem into whether or not you ate a salad for lunch, you're going to have a serious confidence crash when you give in and have a piece or two of cake after dinner. I'm not saying that you shouldn't be proud of making healthy food decisions, but it shouldn't be where your only source of confidence comes from. Doing that can lead to a form of idolatry when we give food the power to determine what kind of life we are going to have.

Healthy and Free Thought

> Your relationship with food can either make or break your journey to health and wellness. When we begin giving food the power to determine what kind of day we are going to have, it becomes a form of idolatry.

Time to Reflect

1. In what ways have I given food power that it shouldn't have had in my life?

_____

_____

_____

2. Do I give food the power to determine what my life or
    relationships look like?

_____

_____

_____

_____

_____

_____

3. How will re-creating my relationship with food help better me on
    my journey?

_____

_____

_____

_____

_____

_____

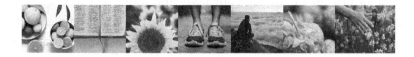

Cultivating Positive Body Image

*You cannot sit back and wait to be happy and
healthy and have a great thought life; you have
to make the choice to make this happen.*
—CAROLINE LEAF

Television, magazines, and the Internet all seem to have their own ideas and perception of how we are supposed to look. Every grocery store is lined with half a dozen magazines that all promise fast weight loss and happiness if you follow their new and improved diet plan, as if you cannot be happy in the body you currently have.

When navigating life in a culture that values perfection, it becomes increasingly easier and easier to break down every part of ourselves that we want to change. Everything from our hair to our eyebrows to our legs to our nails is being constantly picked apart. Trying to keep up gets exhausting!

The truth is, if you cannot learn to love and be comfortable in the body you have now, nothing will change no matter how much weight you lose in the future. Many people think that once they lose *xyz* pounds, then they will have positive body image. However nothing could be further from the truth. There will always, *always* be another trend to follow, body part to tone, and pound to lose.

Creating a positive body image must begin now. You may have spent a lot of your life hating your body and wanting it to change, but remember what we studied about the power of your thoughts. When we choose to hate ourselves, our minds send the message to our body that we are not safe. When we make the conscious decision to love ourselves, our body then gets the message that it is loved and appreciated and begins working in our favor.

The truth is, maybe you aren't at your goal weight or your arms aren't toned just the way you like, but learning to live unapologetically in the body you have is going to build momentum in your journey! Your body will become your best friend, and when you get to the place where you love yourself enough, you will do whatever it takes to see success.

Healthy and Free Thought

> We cannot wait until we have our dream body to be happy. Choosing to love every part of ourselves right now is the key to seeing lasting change and breakthrough in our journey.

Time to Reflect

1. Stand in front of your mirror and take a long look at yourself. Make a list of at least three things that you love. If you have a hard time finding something you love about yourself, ask a friend to show you three things that are beautiful about you.

_____

_____

_____

_____

_____

2.   What three things do you currently love about your body?

3.   What three things do you love about your personality?

4.   Why is it important to begin the process of falling in love with yourself now as opposed to later?

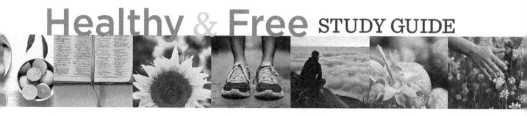

Session 8

The Secret Power of Spirit Health

I once had a student ask me how I handle being a leader when there is a barrage of adversity and attacks attempting to sabotage me. I told her my secret. I deal with these and other stressors by always trying to make sure that I spend time with God before I even leave the house in the morning. God is my rock, so whenever something tries to come against me, I know that I have Him, the solid anchor, holding me steady. Yes, it's true that from time to time you may sway a bit, but your peace comes from knowing that God will always be there to anchor you, to protect you, and to hold you.

Session 8

Video Guide

Keys to Spirit Health

1. Keep _____ with the Holy Spirit.

2. Welcome and pursue _____ with God.

3. Spend time with and _____ to the Holy Spirit.

4. Read your _____.

5. _____ in God's presence.

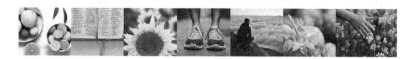

Weekly Health Practice

Pick one verse that the Lord is highlighting to you and write it on a piece of paper or a notecard. Then put the card on your mirror and every morning begin to speak that verse over yourself.

Discussion Questions (25-30 Minutes)

1. How is spiritual starvation just as unhealthy as physical starvation?

2. What are some symptoms of spiritual starvation? Share your own personal signs of spiritual starvation and how you help yourself get back on track.

3. Why is it important that we not only read Scripture silently, but declare it over our lives and ourselves?

4. What improvements should we expect to see when we begin stewarding our spirit health the way God intended?

5. David said in Psalms 1:2 that we are to meditate on His (God's) word day and night. What can we learn from this and why would God find it important for us to meditate on His word?

Activation: Praying the Bible

This is an exercise for you to engage *individually*. In *Healthy and Free*, I wrote about how Stacey and Wesley Campbell taught our church to "pray the Bible." This is a simple concept that includes taking a portion of the Bible and praying it over a certain area or person in your life. Using Psalm 3, begin to pray this over your life. You can personalize it.

For example, when David uses the word *enemies*, you can replace it with whatever battle you seem to be facing—whether it's food addiction, depression, anxiety, etc. After you've personalized and prayed this over yourself, pause for a moment and ask the Holy Spirit to speak to you. Journal what He says in the space below:

_____

_____

_____

_____

_____

_____

_____

_____

_____

_____

_____

_____

_____

_____

_____

_____

_____

_____

_____

_____

_____

_____

_____

_____

_____

_____

_____

_____

_____

_____

Weekly Exercises

Take the time to steward your spirit health. Commit to setting aside ten minutes every day to slow down and focus on creating a connection with the Holy Spirit. Journal what the Holy Spirit is speaking to you about this journey or your life in general.

_____

_____

_____

_____

_____

_____

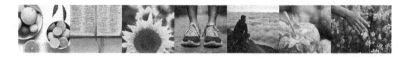

Understanding the Spirit

For then the dust will return to the earth, and
the spirit will return to God who gave it.
—ECCLESIASTES 12:7

We learned a few weeks ago that our soul is our mind. I explained in the book *Healthy and Free* that the soul is what looks earthward and is drawn to earthy things, while the spirit is set on heavenly things. Our spirit is the part of us that communes with God

This may sound ironic considering all we have studied so far, but our spirit is the only part of our being that will continue on for all of eternity. Our bodies will grow old and pass, but our spirits will always live. Because of that, keeping our spirits healthy is perhaps the most important component in overall health and wellness.

If you have ever used spiritual discipline in your life, you may have grown accustomed to meeting and growing your relationship with God. If for some reason you went a few days without spending time with Him, you may have noticed an overt change in your being. Maybe your attitude shifted, you became impatient, over-tired, and stressed. That's because your spirit being was literally starving for its source of nourishment—the Lord. When your spirit becomes starved, your body then reaps the consequences as well once stress and chaos begin to take over. When we keep our spirits healthy, we begin to grow in knowing who we are in the Lord, which then transforms our minds (soul health), which leads to a healthy body.

Keeping your spirit healthy is going to be different for everyone and your spiritual life may change as the Lord guides and leads you through different seasons. For one season, He may be having you focus on studying Scripture or spending time in a particular chapter of the Bible. While in another season you may find that your prayer and worship time will be extended beyond what you've done in that past. It's important to know what season you are in because then you will experience the fullness of what God has for you.

Today, ask the Lord to show you how He wants to spend time with you. If you feel that you are not sure, this week we are going to go through some practical ways to steward your spirit health, so choose the one that most resonates with you.

Healthy and Free Thought

Our relationship with God is what will fuel our spirit with the nourishment it needs. Without the presence of God, we become spiritually starved and on a constant search for something to fulfill us.

Time to Reflect

1. Why is keeping our spirits healthy the most important aspect on this journey to health and wellness?

_____

_____

_____

_____

_____

_____

_____

_____

2. What can I do to make sure I am prioritizing my spirit health and relationship with God?

_____

_____

_____

_____

_____

_____

3. What positive changes will I see take place if I put my spirit health first and foremost?

_____

_____

_____

_____

_____

_____

Day 37

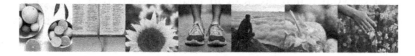

Soaking

Create in me a clean heart, O God, and
renew a right spirit within me.
—Psalm 51:10 ESV

An important part of any relationship is learning when to speak and when to listen. Unfortunately, it's safe to say that the majority of us do not communicate with the audible voice of God as we would a human being. Because of that, it is easy for us to do most of the talking when spending time with God. Just because God doesn't speak an audible language doesn't mean that He doesn't have something to say.

I shared about an encounter I had with the Lord during a trip to Canada. I experienced God in a way that was brand new to me, and I knew that I had to steward this new level of relationship with Him. Upon returning from my trip, I began soaking.

Soaking may be a new concept to some, but it is actually quite simple. Soaking is simply quieting your mind and body while focusing your attention and heart on the Lord. The best way to do this is to lie down in a quiet place where you won't be interrupted. You can use your favorite worship music if you'd like as well. For as long as you need to, just lie in stillness and focus your attention on the beauty and goodness of God. For some, finding an uninterrupted quiet place may be difficult, but even if you only have a few minutes, you will reap great benefits.

Today's challenge for you is to find time to soak. Whether it's in your car on your lunch break or in your bedroom after you've put the kids to bed. Before you soak, take an inventory of how you feel over-all—mind, body, and spirit. Do the same overview after you soak to see if you notice any changes. I'd encourage you to make this exercise a priority if even just for a day. You won't be disappointed that you did.

Healthy and Free Thought

Soaking is a great way to strengthen your spirit man by quieting the world around you and focusing on God.

Time to Reflect

Answer after you complete today's challenge.

1. How did I feel before my soaking session?

    _____

    _____

    _____

    _____

    _____

    _____

2. Were there any noticeable changes in my mind, body, or spirit after I spent time soaking? Explain.

    _____

    _____

    _____

    _____

_____

_____

3. How could taking time out of my day to turn my heart and
    attention toward God change my overall quality of life?

_____

_____

_____

_____

_____

_____

_____

Day 38

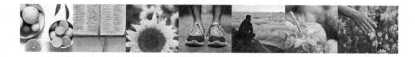

Worship

Worship the Lord your God, and his blessing
will be on your food and water. I will
take away sickness from among you.
—Exodus 23:25 NIV

Worship is perhaps the most intimate communion with God that we can experience here on earth. There is such beauty in being able to raise our hands in worship of Him in the midst of the chaos of everyday life.

Throughout the Bible, we see example after example of the people of God pursuing Him through worship. In 2 Chronicles 20, we read the story of Jehoshaphat receiving news that an army was about to invade his kingdom. He gathered his army together, but instead of waging war on the opposing army, they went forth and worshiped God.

> *After consulting the people, Jehoshaphat appointed men to sing to the Lord and to praise him for the splendor of his holiness as they went out at the head of the army, saying: "Give thanks to the Lord, for his love endures forever." As they began to sing and praise, the Lord set ambushes against the men of Ammon and Moab and Mount Seir who were invading Judah, and they were defeated* (2 Chronicles 20:21-22 NIV).

When the people worshiped, their battle was fought for them by the Lord! This is a beautiful story proclaiming the goodness of God and the power of praising His name. Worship creates an atmosphere that births breakthrough. This is a perfect spiritual weapon especially when embarking on a journey that involves shifting old mindsets and creating new habits.

Today's challenge is to simply worship with abandonment. Release everything that may be coming up against you and give praise to God!

Healthy and Free Thought

Worship creates breakthrough. It brings our spirits into alignment with the goodness and faithfulness of God.

Time to Reflect

Answer after you complete today's challenge.

1. How would worshiping with abandonment look in my life?

_____

_____

_____

_____

_____

_____

2. How would creating a life focused around worship help me on my journey?

_____

_____

_____

_____

_____

_____

_____

3. What changes did I notice after taking time out of my day to
    worship?

_____

_____

_____

_____

_____

_____

_____

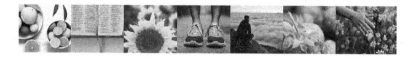

Focused on the Word

This is my comfort and consolation in my affliction:
that Your word has revived me and given me life.
—PSALM 119:50 AMP

The Bible is the only book on the planet that can speak into every situation or season you may face. It brings peace to the anxious heart, hope to the weary, encouragement to the joyful, and life to all. Have you ever found yourself in a difficult season and when you opened your Bible, you felt a noticeable difference in yourself? It's often hard to put that feeling into words, but it is the power of the Word bringing life to your spirit.

Hebrews 4:12 says, *"For the word of God is alive and powerful. It is sharper than the sharpest two-edged sword, cutting between soul and spirit, between joint and marrow. It exposes our innermost thoughts and desires."* Think about that statement for a minute. It is sharper than the *sharpest* two-edged sword. Imagine the amount of breakthrough that we can walk in if we put to use this powerful weapon!

There have been many great people of influence who have left their mark on the world. Jesus, Moses, King David, the apostle Paul, Martin Luther King Jr., and Billy Graham are just a few to mention. Their personal lives may have all looked different, but there is one common trait amongst all of them and that was their passion and dedication to the Word of God.

Today's challenge is to find three scriptures that resonate with your spirit. I want you to write them down and, as you read over them, close your eyes and imagine those words coming to life. Allow yourself to take as much time as you need as allow the Word of God to soak into your spirit.

Healthy and Free Thought

The Bible is known as the living Word of God because it has the ability to bring life to our minds, spirits, and bodies. Meditating and focusing on the Word brings our spirits into alignment with the Spirit of God.

Time to Reflect

Answer after you complete today's challenge.

1. What three verses did I use to speak over my spirit?

   _____

   _____

   _____

2. What noticeable differences did I notice in myself after I meditated on Scripture?

   _____

   _____

   _____

   _____

   _____

   _____

   _____

3. How will I be sure to make Scripture a priority in my day-to-day life?

_____

_____

_____

_____

_____

_____

_____

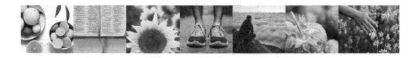

Enjoying Your Time with God

You will show me the way of life, granting me the joy of
your presence and the pleasures of living with you forever.
—PSALM 16:11

By now, you may have begun exploring new ways to bring life and health to your spirit. At times you may have felt uncomfortable and stretched, but hopefully you were able to encounter God in a new and beautiful way.

Part of the Christian walk is allowing ourselves to be uncomfortable and stretched in certain areas of our faith; however, when it comes to spending time with God, it doesn't always have to be that way. God loves us unconditionally and loves spending time with us doing the things that we love to do.

Remember, He created us in His image. So the things that bring you joy and life also bring Him joy and life. Spending time with Him doesn't have to always look like going to a church worship service or reading two chapters of the Bible in one sitting. It could look like getting out a blank canvas and painting while keeping your spirit aware of the Presence of God around you. It could look like spending time in the kitchen experimenting and cooking a meal for family and friends. You can also encounter God while singing, playing an instrument, working out, etc.!

God is not limited to a Bible reading or a worship song. Keep in mind that He wants to encounter you more than you want to encounter Him.

Healthy and Free Thought

God not only wants to spend time with us, He *likes* to spend time with us. Stewarding our spirit's health can look like spending time with God doing the things that we love to do.

Time to Reflect

1. What are some things I find joy doing that I can invite the Holy Spirit's Presence to join me while I do them?

2. Knowing that God wants to encounter me more than I want to encounter Him, how does that change the way I pursue the Presence of God?

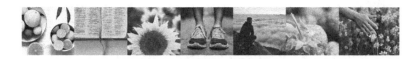

Answer Key

Session 1: Find Your Why

1. why

2. Partner

3. baby

4. option

5. long

6. lifestyle

7. mind

8. hope

9. grace

10. keep

11. own

Session 2: The Secret Power of Soul Health

1. love

2. permission

3. Talk

4. Encourage

5. says

6. Laugh

7.   good

8.   arrest

9.   declarations

Session 3: The Body, Soul and Spirit Connection

Responsibility

Session 4: The Power of Sleep and Water

1.   70

2.   dehydrate

3.   alkalizes

4.   energize

1.   sun

2.   magnesium

Session 5: Movement

1.   move

2.   protect

3.   lifestyle

Session 8: The Secret Power of Spirit Health

6.   union

7.   encounters

8.   talk

9.   Bible

10. Soak

THE SUPERNATURAL POWER
OF A TRANSFORMED MIND
CURRICULUM

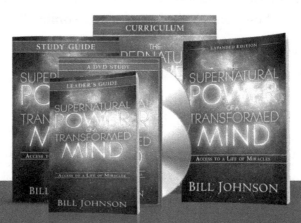

"A WAKE-UP CALL TO THE 'GREATER
THINGS THAN THESE SHALL YOU DO'
PROMISE OF JESUS." - RANDY CLARK

In *Supernatural Power of a Transformed Mind*, Pastor Bill Johnson delivers powerful and practical teaching, revealing how you were designed to bring heaven to Earth and how it all starts with your thought life.

Your access to a lifestyle of signs, wonders, and miracles starts by changing the way you think. When your mind is transformed, heaven becomes more than a place you go to one day—it becomes the supernatural power that you release wherever you go today!

INCLUDED IN THIS CURRICULUM:

DVD Study and Leader's Guide • Study Guide • *Supernatural Power of a Transformed Mind* Book

YOUR HEALTHY & FREE LIFESTYLE IS JUST ONE DECISION AWAY...

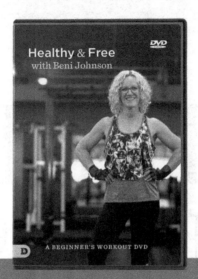

EXERCISE.

In this workout DVD, Beni Johnson gives you fun, easy-to-follow exercises that leave you without excuse.

She makes working out so easy and fun that no matter how busy your schedule is, you can still make one of the most important investments of all: a healthy lifestyle!

Beni gives you over two hours of exciting and enjoyable workouts that will show you...

- How to exercise anywhere... from the comfort of your own home to the scenic environment of a park
- How to comfortably and effectively use equipment in your home
- How to confidently use gym machines to maximize your workout impact and effectiveness

Once you begin the journey and start feeling the results in your body, you will make working out a regular part of your schedule that will set you on course for a lifetime of living healthy and free!

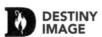